The Endocrine System at a Glance

The Endocrine System at a Glance

Ben Greenstein

BA (Hons) PhD
Senior Visiting Research Fellow
Pain Management Unit
Royal Free School of Medicine
London
UK

Diana Wood

MA MD FRCP
Director of Medical Education and Clinical Dean
University of Cambridge School of Clinical Medicine
Clinical School
Addenbrooke's Hospital
Cambridge
UK

Third edition

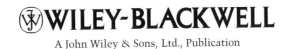

A John Wiley & Sons, Ltd., Publication

This edition first published 2011 © 2011 by Ben Greenstein and Diana Wood
First edition 1994
Second edition 2006

Wiley-Blackwell is an imprint of John Wiley & Sons, formed by the merger of Wiley's global
Scientific, Technical and Medical business with Blackwell Publishing.

Registered office: John Wiley & Sons, Ltd, The Atrium, Southern Gate, Chichester, West Sussex,
  PO19 8SQ, UK

Editorial offices: 9600 Garsington Road, Oxford, OX4 2DQ, UK
  The Atrium, Southern Gate, Chichester, West Sussex, PO19 8SQ, UK
  111 River Street, Hoboken, NJ 07030–5774, USA

For details of our global editorial offices, for customer services and for information about how
to apply for permission to reuse the copyright material in this book please see our website at
www.wiley.com/wiley-blackwell.

Library of Congress Cataloging-in-Publication Data
Greenstein, Ben, 1941-
  The endocrine system at a glance / Ben Greenstein, Diana Wood. – 3rd ed.
    p. ; cm. – (At a glance series)
  Includes index.
  ISBN-13: 978-1-4443-3215-5 (pbk. : alk. paper)
  ISBN-10: 1-4443-3215-5
  1. Endocrinology. I. Wood, Diana F. II. Title. III. Series: At a glance series (Oxford, England)
    [DNLM: 1. Endocrine Glands–physiology. 2. Endocrine Glands–
physiopathology. 3. Endocrine System Diseases. 4. Hormones–secretion. WK 100]
  QP187.G834 2011
  612.4–dc22

                                                2011007204

A catalogue record for this book is available from the British Library.

Set in 9.5/12 pt Times-Roman by Toppan Best-set Premedia Limited

Contents

Preface to the Third Edition

The third edition of this book is again co-authored by Ben Greenstein and Diana Wood, a clinical endocrinologist. The book aims to relate basic endocrine sciences to the clinical background and presentations of disease and in keeping with the overall philosophy of the *At a Glance* series, and strives to present data in a varied way that facilitates rapid assimilation of the information. The book is aimed at undergraduate medical students, primarily in the early part of their course, although as a handy and accessible reference book and revision tool it should also be a useful source of information for clinical medical students and junior doctors. *The Endocrine System at a Glance*, as the name implies, does not claim to replace comprehensive textbooks; rather it serves as a concise guide and revision aid to this fascinating branch of clinical science and medicine. A new addition to the third edition is the presentation of revision questions relating to each chapter.

The authors have striven to present the data clearly and accurately, and every effort has been made to include information that is up-to-date at the time of going to press. We make no claim to infallibility, however, and if readers spot ambiguities, factual inaccuracies or typographical errors, we should be most grateful for feedback and for suggestions which will improve the book and the presentation of the information.

It remains for us to thank the many students and colleagues who have read and commented on the book while in draft form. It has been a pleasure to work with the staff at Wiley-Blackwell, and in particular Karen Moore and Beth Bishop, whose patience and guidance is much appreciated.

Ben Greenstein
Diana Wood
London and Cambridge

Preface to the First Edition

Endocrinology at a Glance published 1994

Endocrinology at a Glance is intended to be just that. It has been designed and written so that the diagrams and text complement each other, and both are to be consulted. The emphasis has been on the diagrams, and words have been kept to a minimum.

The book has been produced to provide as comprehensive an overview of the subject as any medical or science undergraduate student will need in order to pass and pass well an examination in basic endocrinology. In addition, it is hoped that *Endocrinology at a Glance* will be useful to students of clinical endocrinology who need to refer rapidly to the mechanisms underlying the subject. The book is not presented as an alternative to the several excellent textbooks of endocrinology, which serve as useful reference texts, and some of which have been used during the writing of this book.

Every attempt has been made to present the data accurately and to provide the most up-to-date and reliable information available. When speculative data are given, their fragility has been indicated. Nevertheless, every writer, especially this one, is human and if the reader spots errors or a lack of clarity, or has any suggestions to improve or add to the presentation, this feedback will be gratefully appreciated and acknowledged.

I should like to thank the many undergraduate, medical, dental and science students who have scrutinized and used the diagrams, or similar ones, over the years, and whose criticisms have helped to make them more useful. I should like to thank Elizabeth Bridges, Kay Chan, Yacoub Dhaher, Munther Khamashta and Adam Greenstein for commentating on some of the work. It has been a pleasure working with the staff of Blackwell Science Ltd, and particularly Dr Stuart Taylor and Emma Lynch, whose friendly encouragement and advice cheered me on.

Ben Greenstein
London 1994

1 Introduction

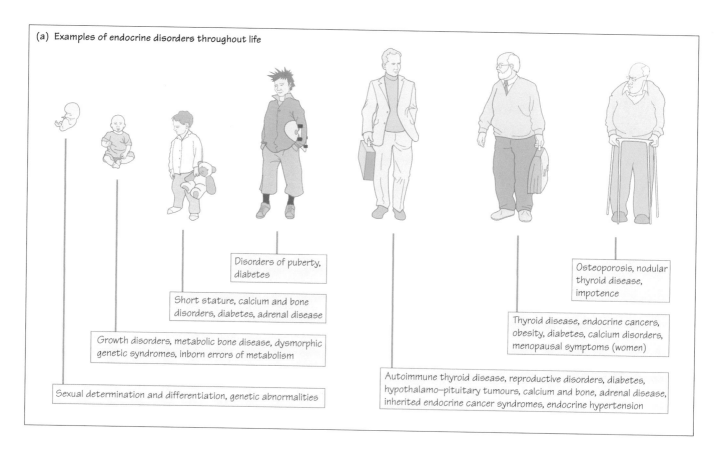

(a) Examples of endocrine disorders throughout life

Disorders of puberty, diabetes

Short stature, calcium and bone disorders, diabetes, adrenal disease

Growth disorders, metabolic bone disease, dysmorphic genetic syndromes, inborn errors of metabolism

Sexual determination and differentiation, genetic abnormalities

Osteoporosis, nodular thyroid disease, impotence

Thyroid disease, endocrine cancers, obesity, diabetes, calcium disorders, menopausal symptoms (women)

Autoimmune thyroid disease, reproductive disorders, diabetes, hypothalamo–pituitary tumours, calcium and bone, adrenal disease, inherited endocrine cancer syndromes, endocrine hypertension

Clinical background

Endocrinology is the study of endocrine hormones and of the organs involved in endocrine hormone release. Classically, hormones have been described as chemical messengers, released and having their actions at distant sites. It is now clear, however, that there is a close relationship between hormones and other factors such as neurotransmitters and growth factors acting in a paracrine or autocrine fashion. Hormones are essential for the maintenance of normal physiological function and hormonal disorders occur at all stages of human life. Clinical endocrinologists thus look after patients of all ages and with a very wide range of disorders (Fig. 1a).

The principal endocrine glands

The brain is the controller of the nervous system, but it is also one of the most important endocrine glands. Specialized nerve cells, notably in the hypothalamus, synthesize hormones which are transported along the axon to the nerve terminal. Here they are released into the portal blood system, which carries them to the pituitary gland. In some cases, the axon of the neuroendocrine cell projects down to the pituitary cell itself. The principal hypothalamic neurohormones are:

1 corticotrophin-releasing hormone (CRH), controls the release of ACTH;

2 dopamine inhibits prolactin release;

3 growth-hormone-releasing hormone (GHRH) causes growth hormone release;

4 somatostatin inhibits growth hormone release;

5 gonadotrophin-releasing hormone (GnRH) causes luteinizing hormone (LH) and follicle-stimulating hormone (FSH) release;

6 thyrotrophin-releasing hormone (TRH) causes thyroid-stimulating hormone (TSH) release;

7 oxytocin causes milk ejection and contraction of the uterus in labour – it is synthesized in the hypothalamus and is stored in and released from the posterior pituitary gland;

8 vasopressin (antidiuretic hormone, ADH) promotes water reabsorption from the kidney tubules – it is synthesized in the hypothalamus, and stored in and released from the posterior pituitary gland.

The pituitary gland is composed of two lobes, anterior and posterior, which arise from different embryological origins – the anterior originates from the embryonic oral cavity and the posterior from the base of the brain (i.e. a neural origin). The two lobes become closely apposed to each other to form the pituitary gland. Humans have a non-functional **intermediate lobe**, which is much larger in some other animals. The principal hormones of the pituitary are:

1 **anterior:**

(a) **corticotrophin** (adrenocorticotrophic hormone; ACTH) releases glucocorticoids and other steroids from the adrenal cortex;

(b) **follicle-stimulating hormone** (FSH) promotes spermatogenesis in males and ovarian follicular maturation in females;

(c) **luteinizing hormone** (LH) promotes testosterone synthesis in males and causes ovarian follicular rupture and ovulation in females;

(d) **prolactin** (PRL) promotes lactation and may have an immunomodulatory role in non-lactating females and males;

(e) **thyrotrophin** (thyroid-stimulating hormone; TSH) promotes thyroid hormone production and release from the thyroid gland;

(f) **growth hormone** (also called somatotrophin; GH) promotes muscle and skeletal growth.

2 **posterior:**

(a) **oxytocin** causes milk ejection and contraction of the uterus in labour;

(b) **vasopressin** (antidiuretic hormone, ADH) promotes water reabsorption from the renal tubules.

The thyroid gland is situated just in front of the trachea in humans. The thyroid-hormone-producing cells are arranged in follicles, and concentrate iodine which is used for the synthesis of the thyroid hormone. The circulating hormones are **thyroxine (T_4)** and **tri-iodothyronine (T_3)**. **The parathyroid glands** are embedded in the thyroid, and produce **parathyroid hormone** (parathormone; PTH). PTH is important in the control of calcium and phosphate metabolism. **The parafollicular cells** are in the thyroid, scattered between the follicles. They produce **calcitonin**, which inhibits bone calcium resorption.

The adrenal glands are situated just above the kidneys, and are composed of an outer layer, or cortex, and an inner layer, or medulla (a modified ganglion). The hormones produced are:

1 **cortex:**

(a) **glucocorticoids**, principally cortisol in humans, are involved in carbohydrate metabolism and the response to stress;

(b) **mineralocorticoids**, principally aldosterone, control electrolyte balance;

(c) **androgens**, principally testosterone, dehydroepiandrostenedione sulphate (DHEAS) and 17-hydroxyprogesterone, modulate secondary sexual characteristics and have anabolic effects.

2 **medulla:**

(a) **epinephrine** modulates cardiovascular and metabolic response to stress;

(b) **norepinephrine**, principally a neurotransmitter in the peripheral sympathetic nervous system;

(c) **dopamine**, a neurotransmitter in the autonomic nervous system.

The endocrine pancreas consists of islet cells scattered in the larger exocrine pancreas, which lies posteriorly in the upper abdomen. ('Exocrine' refers to glands which have ducts, and which are not covered in this book.) The endocrine pancreas secretes:

1 **insulin**, which regulates glucose and lipid metabolism;

2 **glucagon**, a counter-regulatory hormone to insulin that elevates blood glucose;

3 **somatostatin**, which regulates gastrointestinal motility;

4 **pancreatic polypeptide**, which regulates gastrointestinal secretion.

The ovary is the major female reproductive gland, and produces:

1 **estrogens**, which regulate reproductive function and secondary sexual characteristics;

2 **progesterone**, which stimulates endometrial vascularization and maintains pregnancy;

3 **relaxin**, a polypeptide also found in the placenta and uterus, which may be important in parturition by softening the cervix and relaxing the pelvic ligaments;

4 **inhibin**, which inhibits FSH production.

The placenta is the organ of pregnancy serving the developing fetus. Hormones produced by the placenta include:

1 **chorionic gonadotrophin** (CG; hCG; h = human) which maintains placental progesterone synthesis;

2 **placental lactogen** (PL);

3 **estriol**, the major form of estrogen secreted by the placenta;

4 **progesterone** which maintains the reproductive organs in pregnancy;

5 **relaxin.**

The testis is the major male reproductive gland, producing:

1 **testosterone** which controls reproductive function and secondary sexual characteristics;

2 **inhibin**, which inhibits FSH secretion;

3 **Müllerian inhibiting hormone** (MIH), a fetal hormone which dedifferentiates the Müllerian duct.

The gastrointestinal tract (GIT) is the largest endocrine organ and produces several autocrine, paracrine and endocrine hormones including:

1 **cholecystokinin** (CCK);

2 **gastric inhibitory peptide** (GIP);

3 **gastrin;**

4 **neurotensin;**

5 **secretin;**

6 **substance P;**

7 **vasoactive intestinal peptide** (VIP).

Adipocytes produce the peptide hormone **leptin** which is important in the control of feeding and energy expenditure.

The kidney produces hormones involved in the control of blood pressure and in erythropoiesis. **Renin** cleaves angiotensinogen to angiotensin I in the kidney and plasma. **Erythropoietin** stimulates production of red blood cells in the marrow.

The skin, liver and kidney produce vitamin D which has certain endocrine functions.

The heart produces atrial natriuretic peptide. **Circulating blood elements**, including macrophages, produce peptides such as the cytokines, which are involved in immune function.

The pineal gland is situated in the brain and is involved with rhythms, for example the reproductive rhythms of animals which breed seasonally. Its role in humans is not known for certain. The pineal gland produces **melatonin**.

Readers should be aware that putative endocrine hormones continue to be reported.

2 Chemical transmission

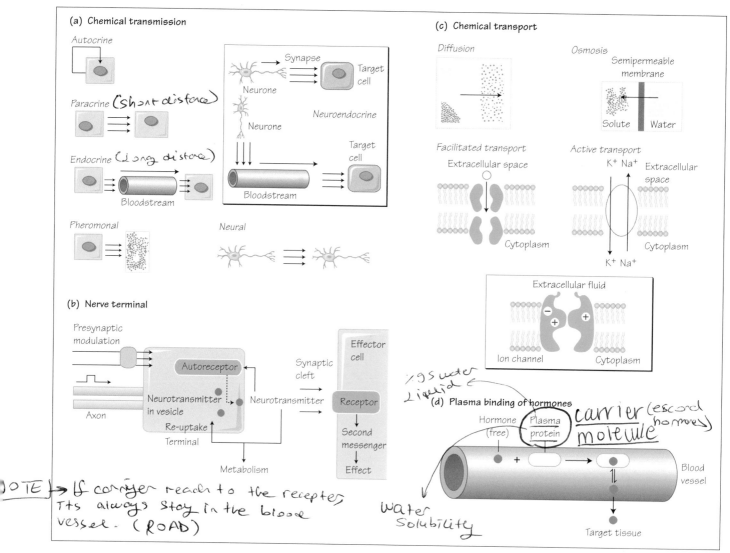

(a) Chemical transmission

Autocrine

Paracrine (short distance)

Endocrine (long distance)
Bloodstream

Synapse → Target cell
Neurone
Neurone → Neuroendocrine
Target cell
Bloodstream

Pheromonal

Neural

(b) Nerve terminal

Presynaptic modulation

Autoreceptor
Neurotransmitter in vesicle → Neurotransmitter
Axon
Re-uptake
Terminal
Metabolism

Synaptic cleft

Effector cell
Receptor
Second messenger
Effect

(c) Chemical transport

Diffusion

Osmosis
Semipermeable membrane
Solute   Water

Facilitated transport
Extracellular space

Cytoplasm

Active transport
K^+ Na^+ Extracellular space

Cytoplasm
K^+ Na^+

Extracellular fluid

Ion channel   Cytoplasm

(handwritten) i9s water Liquid ←
(d) Plasma binding of hormones
Hormone (free)   Plasma protein — *carrier (escort hormones) molecule*

(handwritten) water solubility

Blood vessel

Target tissue

(handwritten) NOTE → If carrier reach to the recepter Its always stay in the blood vessel. (ROAD)

Classification of endocrine hormones

Hormones are chemical messengers. They may be classified several ways (Fig. 2a):

1 Autocrine: acting on the cells that synthesized them; for example insulin-like growth factor (IGF-1) which stimulates cell division in the cell which produced it.

2 Paracrine: acting on neighbouring cells. An example is insulin, secreted by pancreatic b cells and affecting secretion of glucagon by pancreatic a cells.

3 Endocrine: acting on cells or organs to which they are carried in the bloodstream or through another aqueous ducting system, such as lymph. Examples include insulin, estradiol and cortisol.

4 Neuroendocrine: this is really paracrine or endocrine, except that the hormones are synthesized in a nerve cell (neurone) which releases the hormone adjacent to the target cell (paracrine), or releases it into the bloodstream, which carries it to the target cell, for example from the hypothalamus to the anterior pituitary gland through the portal system.

5 Neural: this is neurotransmission, when a chemical is released by one neurone and acts on an adjacent neurone (Fig. 2b). These chemicals are termed neurotransmitters. Neurotransmitters produce virtually instantaneous effects, for example acetylcholine, whereas some chemicals have a slower onset but longer lasting effect on the target organ, and are termed **neuromodulators**, for example certain opioids.

6 Pheromonal transmission is the release of volatile hormones, called pheromones, into the atmosphere, where they are transmitted to another individual and are recognized as an olfactory signal.

Basic principles of neurotransmission

When the nerve impulse arrives at the terminal, it triggers a calcium-dependent fusion of neurotransmitter packets or vesicles with the nerve terminal plasma membrane (Fig. 2b), followed by release of the neurotransmitter into the gap, or synapse, between the nerve cells. The neurotransmitters and neuromodulators bind to specific plasma membrane receptors, which

 The Endocrine System at a Glance, 3rd edition. © Ben Greenstein and Diana Wood. Published 2011 by Blackwell Publishing Ltd.

transmit the information that the neurotransmitter has brought to the receiving cell by means of other membrane proteins and intracellular 'second messengers'. The neurotransmitters are inactivated by enzymes or taken up into the nerve that released them and metabolized. The release of the neurotransmitter may be modulated and limited by: (i) autoreceptors on the nerve terminal from which it was released, so that further release of the neurotransmitter is inhibited; and (ii) by presynaptic inhibition, when another neurone synapses with the nerve terminal.

Chemical transport

The movement of chemicals between cells and organs is usually tightly controlled.

Diffusion is the movement of molecules in a fluid phase, in random thermal (Brownian) motion (Fig. 2c). If two solutions containing the same chemical, one concentrated and the other relatively dilute, are separated by a membrane which is completely permeable and passive, the concentrations of the chemical on either side of the membrane will eventually end up being the same through simple diffusion of solutes. This is because there are many molecules of the chemical on the concentrated side, and therefore a statistically greater probability of movement from the more concentrated side to the more dilute side of the membrane. Eventually, when the concentrations are equal on both sides, the net change on either side becomes zero. Lipophilic molecules such as ethyl alcohol and the steroids, for example estradiol, appear to diffuse freely across all biological membranes.

Facilitated transport is the transport of chemicals across membranes by carrier proteins. The process does not require energy and cannot, therefore, transport chemicals against a concentration gradient. The numbers of transporter proteins may be under hormonal control. Glucose is carried into the cell by transporter proteins (see Chapter 39) whose numbers are increased by insulin.

Active transport uses energy in the form of adenosine triphosphate (ATP) or other metabolic fuels. Therefore chemicals can be transported across the membrane against a concentration gradient, and the transport process can be interrupted by metabolic poisons.

Ion channels mediate active transport, and consist of proteins containing charged amino acids that may form activation and inactivation 'gates'. Ion channels may be activated by receptors, or by voltage changes through the cell membrane. Channels of the ion Ca^{2+} can be activated by these two methods.

Osmosis is the passive movement of water through a semipermeable membrane, from a compartment of low solute concentration to one which has a greater concentration of the solute. ('Solute' refers to the chemical which is dissolved in the 'solvent', usually water in biological tissues.) Cells will shrink or swell depending on the concentrations of the solutes on either side of the membrane.

Phagocytosis and pinocytosis are both examples of endocytosis. Substances can enter the cell without having to pass through the cell membrane. Phagocytosis is the ingestion or 'swallowing' of a solid particle by a cell, while pinocytosis is the ingestion of fluid. Receptor-mediated endocytosis is the ingestion of specifically recognized substances by coated pits. These are parts of the membrane which are coated with specific membrane proteins, for example clathrin. **Exocytosis** is the movement of substances, such as hormones, out of the cell. Chemicals which are stored in the small vesicles or packets are secreted or released from the cell in which they are stored by exocytosis, when the vesicle fuses with the membrane.

Hormone transport in blood. When hormones are secreted into the blood, many are immediately bound to plasma proteins (Fig. 2d). The proteins may recognize the hormone specifically and bind it with high affinity and specificity, for example the binding of sex hormones by sex hormone-binding globulin (SHBG). Other proteins, such as albumin, also bind many hormones, including thyroid hormone and the sex hormones, with much lower affinity. Equilibrium is set up between the free and bound hormone, so that a fixed proportion of the hormone travels free and unbound, while most is carried bound. It is currently believed that only the free fraction of the hormone is physiologically active and available to the tissues and for metabolism. When a hormone is bound to plasma proteins it is physiologically inactive and is also protected from metabolic enzymes in organs such as the liver. Some drugs, such as aspirin, can displace other substances such as anticoagulants from their binding sites, which in the case of anticoagulants may cause haemorrhage.

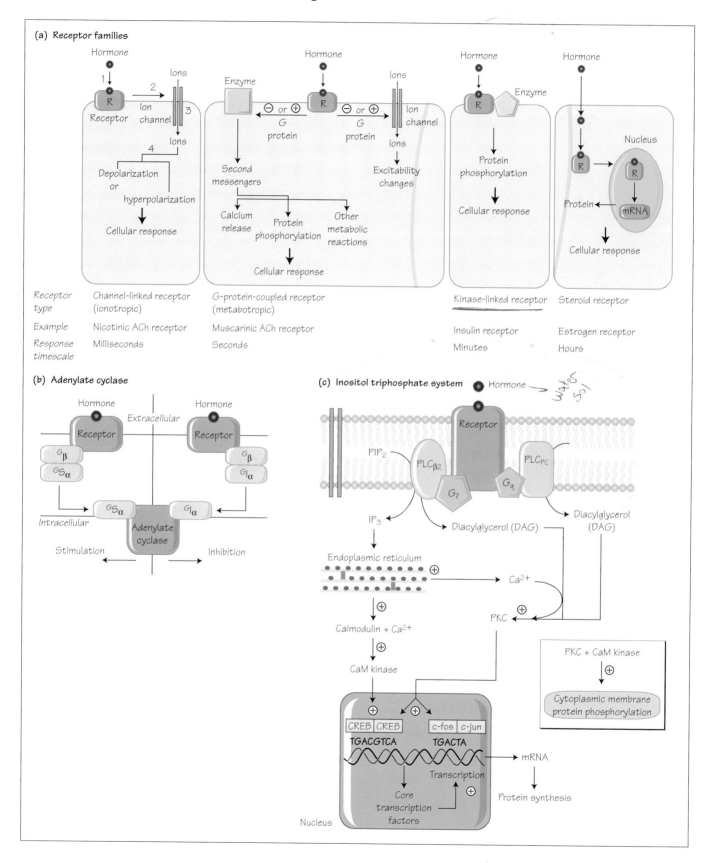

(a) Receptor families

Receptor type	Channel-linked receptor (ionotropic)	G-protein-coupled receptor (metabotropic)	Kinase-linked receptor	Steroid receptor
Example	Nicotinic ACh receptor	Muscarinic ACh receptor	Insulin receptor	Estrogen receptor
Response timescale	Milliseconds	Seconds	Minutes	Hours

(b) Adenylate cyclase

(c) Inositol triphosphate system

Clinical background

Acromegaly is usually caused by anterior pituitary gland tumours which secrete growth hormone. In 30 to 40% of cases, the tumour is thought to arise due to a somatic mutation affecting transmembrane signalling mechanisms. The stimulatory G-protein Gs is involved in signal transduction at the growth hormone releasing hormone receptor. Mutation of the α-subunit of Gs into the *gsp* oncogene prolongs the activation phase of the G-protein system, allowing unrestrained hormone synthesis and cell division. The distinctive clinical features of acromegaly and development of the pituitary tumour follow.

Introduction

Hormones interact with target cells through a primary interaction with receptors which recognize the hormones selectively. There are several different receptor systems, which vary in mechanism and timing (Fig. 3a). Charged ions such as peptides and neurotransmitters bind to receptors on the cell membrane. This causes a conformational change in other membrane proteins, which activate enzymes inside the cell, resulting in, for example, the synthesis of 'second messengers', which activate phosphorylating enzymes.

Uncharged molecules, such as the steroid hormones diffuse into the cell and bind to intracellular receptors (see Chapter 4). The hormone–receptor complex binds to specific hormone response elements (HRE) on the DNA; the result is that RNA and protein synthesis are altered. The cell will react faster to peptide hormones and neurotransmitters than it will to steroid hormones, which work through relatively slow changes in protein synthesis. Nevertheless, membrane receptors have been discovered for steroid hormones, although the significance of these is not yet clear.

Membrane receptors

Three regions can be distinguished in membrane receptors: the extracellular; the membrane-spanning; and the intracellular domains. The extracellular N-terminal domain has the hormone-binding domain, and also has glycosylation sites. The extracellular domain that binds the receptor is often rich in cysteine residues, which form rigid pockets in which the hormone is bound. The transmembrane region consists of one or more segments, made up of hydrophobic (uncharged) amino acids, arranged helically, whose role may include the anchoring of the receptor in the membrane. Different subunits within the membrane may be held together by means of disulphide linkages (e.g. the insulin receptor, Chapter 39). The intracellular domain is the effector region of the receptor, which may be linked with another membrane protein system, a set of enzymes which are guanosine triphosphatases (GTPases). The β-adrenergic receptor is an example of a G-protein-linked receptor. Another class, which includes the insulin receptor, has the intracellular domain as a tyrosine protein kinase. The intracellular region may also have a regulatory tyrosine or serine/ threonine phosphorylation site.

Second messengers

G protein linked receptors. These are protein receptors in the cell membrane, with an extracellular domain and an intracellular domain. The peptide chain that forms the protein always spans the membrane. When the hormone binds to the extracellular domain, this causes a change in shape of the receptor. This causes the intracellular domain to activate G proteins. G proteins have three main parts: an a subunit, a b subunit and a g subunit. When activated, firstly the a subunit substitutes a GDP molecule for a GTP molecule. This results in the activation of the G proteins. They can be either stimulatory or inhibitory, that is they can cause an increased level of enzyme activity or a decreased level of activity in the second messenger systems. Mutations of G proteins can occur and may result in disease (see Clinical scenario above).

Adenylate cyclase system. The hormone binds to the receptor, which activates a membrane G protein, which moves to the receptor (Fig. 3b). In the inactive state, the G protein binds GDP, which is exchanged for GTP, and a subunit of the G protein activates adenylate cyclase to convert ATP to the second messenger cyclic AMP. Adenylate cyclase is situated on the plasma membrane, but does not itself bind the hormone. Once formed in the cytoplasm, cAMP activates the catalytic subunit of a specific protein kinase (PKA), which forms part of a cascade of intracellular phosphorylations resulting in the cellular response. Since just one molecule of hormone can result in the production of many molecules of cAMP, this is a very efficient means of amplifying the receptor–hormone interaction. Once formed, cAMP is rapidly broken down by the enzyme phosphodiesterase. An example of a hormone operating through adenylate cyclase is epinephrine, through the adrenergic β-receptor.

Hormones can produce inhibitory effects on a cell, and this may be achieved through the fact that some G proteins, such as G_I, may inhibit adenylate cyclase, thus inhibiting the formation of cAMP. An example of this mechanism in action is the inhibition of adenylate cyclase through the binding of norepinephrine to the α-2-receptor on the presynaptic nerve terminal.

Inositol triphosphate system. In this system, the hormone–receptor–G-protein complex interaction triggers the membrane enzyme phospholipase C (PLC), which catalyses the hydrolysis of phosphoinositol (PIP2) to two important metabolites, inositol triphosphate (IP3) and diacylglycerol (DAG; Fig. 3c). IP3 generates, from the endoplasmic endothelium, increased free Ca^{2+}, which together with DAG promotes the activation and migration to the membrane of the enzyme protein kinase C (PKC). PKC may also be mobilized through the entry of Ca^{2+} into the cell. Examples of hormones and neurotransmitters which activate the system are **epinephrine** acting on α-1 receptors and **acetylcholine** on muscarinic cholinergic receptors. These systems are important clinically since they provide substantial numbers of possible targets for drugs.

Receptor antagonists

Receptor antagonism is an important aspect of endocrinology and drug use generally, not only in terms of the study of the hormone–receptor interaction, but also in therapeutic terms, since antagonists play a large part in the treatment of endocrine disease. The molecule which binds to the receptor and elicits the normal cellular response is termed the **agonist**. The ligand which binds, but elicits no response, is the **antagonist**. Antagonists act at the membrane in different ways. For example the β-receptor blocker propranolol competes with epinephrine at its binding site. The anticonvulsant phenytoin blocks ion channels.

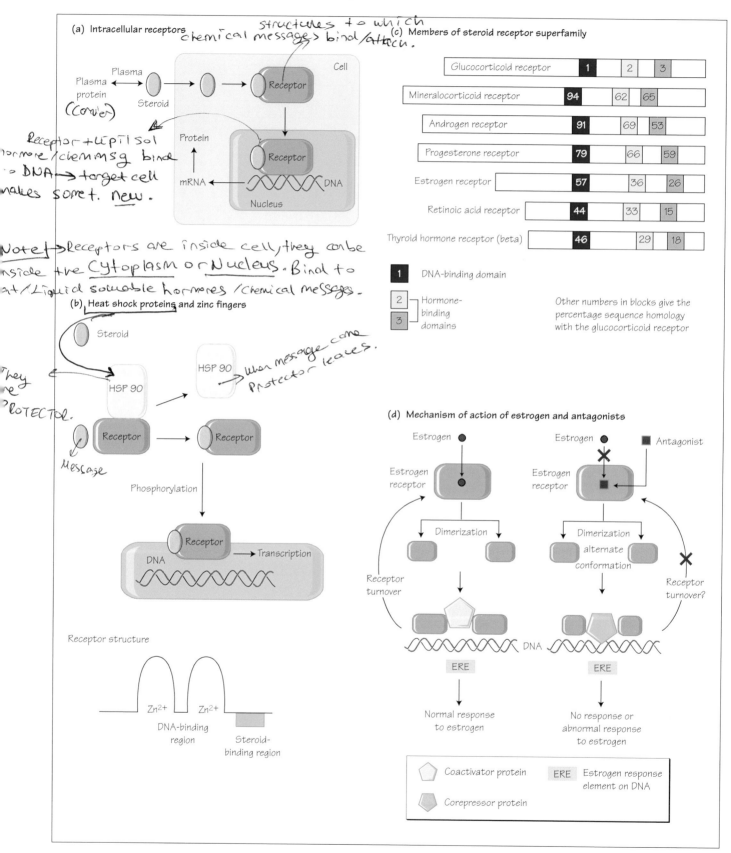

(a) Intracellular receptors

Handwritten annotations:
structures to which chemical message> bind/attach.

Receptor + leptisol hormone/chem msg bind to DNA → target cell makes somet. new.

Note! → Receptors are inside cell, they can be inside the Cytoplasm or Nucleus. Bind to at/Liquid soluble hormones/chemical messages.

They re PROTECTOR.

Message

When message come Protector leaves.

(b) Heat shock proteins and zinc fingers

(c) Members of steroid receptor superfamily

	DNA-binding domain (1)	Hormone-binding domain (2)	(3)
Glucocorticoid receptor	1	2	3
Mineralocorticoid receptor	94	62	65
Androgen receptor	91	69	53
Progesterone receptor	79	66	59
Estrogen receptor	57	36	26
Retinoic acid receptor	44	33	15
Thyroid hormone receptor (beta)	46	29	18

1 DNA-binding domain

2 Hormone-binding domains
3

Other numbers in blocks give the percentage sequence homology with the glucocorticoid receptor

(d) Mechanism of action of estrogen and antagonists

Coactivator protein

ERE Estrogen response element on DNA

Corepressor protein

Clinical background

Estrogen stimulates the proliferation of breast cancer tissue and exposure to estrogens may be important in the pathogenesis of this disease. During the treatment of women with breast cancer it is routine practice to establish the presence (ER +ve) or absence (ER -ve) of estrogen receptors in cancer cells. Women who have ER +ve tumours are more likely to respond to endocrine manipulation following surgery and/or chemotherapy (50–60% response rate in ER +ve cancers, 5–10% in ER –ve tumours). The most commonly used endocrine therapy is the drug tamoxifen which has estrogen-antagonist effects in the breast, probably mediated by the recruitment of corepressors for estrogen receptor action. It produces a significant fall in tumour recurrence and death rates for women with ER +ve disease, irrespective of age. The possible use of tamoxifen and the newer, selective estrogen receptor modulator drugs (SERMs, e.g. raloxifene, toremifine) for the prevention of breast cancer are under investigation. Trastuzumab, a humanized IgG1 against human epidermal growth factor receptor-2 (HER-2+), is now used to treat early breast cancer that overexpresses HER-2.

Intracellular receptors

Lipophilic hormones, such as steroids and the thyroid hormones, pass easily through the plasma membrane into the cell, where they combine with specific receptor proteins (Fig. 4a). In the inactive state, for the subfamily of glucocorticoid, progesterone, estrogen and androgen receptors, the receptor is bound to a heat shock protein (HSP 90; Fig. 4b).

When the hormone binds to the receptor, the HSP dissociates from it, the receptors form homodimers and the hormone–receptor complex binds to DNA at specific sites, termed hormone response elements (HREs), which lie upstream from transcription initiation sites. Transcription and subsequent protein synthesis are altered. The thyroid hormone and retinoic acid receptors are not associated with HSPs in their inactive state, and are able to associate with their response elements on the DNA in the absence of the hormones, and act as transcription inhibitors (see also below). Activation of receptors expressing the actions of the hormones appears to be achieved through phosphorylation, although at present this process is poorly understood.

Nature of the steroid receptor

The steroid receptors form part of a larger 'superfamily' of nuclear DNA-binding receptors, including androgen, estrogen, glucocorticoid, thyroid and vitamin D receptors (Fig. 4c). They all have two main regions, a hydrophobic hormone-binding region and a DNA-binding region, which consists of two 'zinc fingers', rich in cysteine and basic amino acids. The structures of the receptors are known. Region 1 is the DNA-binding region, and is the most conserved among the members of the receptor family, in that it has a high sequence homology from receptor to receptor, as shown in Fig. 4c. It is thought that the first zinc finger determines the specificity of the binding of the receptor to DNA, while the second finger stabilizes the receptor to its response element of the DNA. Regions 2 and 3 of the receptors determine the hormone specificity of binding, and are not well conserved among the different receptors.

Estrogen receptors

Two distinct, main receptor forms have been discovered, called ER-α and ER-β respectively. They have different affinities for estradiol and different anatomical distribution. For example only ER-α has been found in the liver, and ER-β is the predominant form in prostate. These differences may account, in part, for the wide diversity of estrogen action in different tissues and under different physiological and pathological states. It has been found, for example, that in healthy ovarian tissue the β form predominates, but in ovarian cancer the a form predominates. It is possible that the β form somehow regulates the activity of the α form. The α and β forms have several nuclear coactivators and repressors, and their activity depends also on their rates of turnover.

Estrogen receptor antagonists have found a powerful use in the prevention and treatment of breast cancer (see **Clinical scenario** above). These compounds interfere with the processing of the normal intracellular hormone–receptor interaction. This can occur at one or more of several sites (Fig. 4d). The receptor itself may be blocked or post-receptor-binding events, for example receptor dimerization, receptor turnover or mRNA or protein synthesis, may be inhibited. Examples of estrogen receptor blockers are the **SERMS** (selective estrogen receptor modulators) such as tamoxifen, raloxifene and toremifene. These are interesting because they appear to act as agonists in some tissues such as bone and liver cells, and may therefore be important preventive measures for reducing the rate of development of osteoporosis and for lowering blood cholesterol. SERMS may act by activating as yet unidentified coactivators or corepressors and may modulate estrogen receptor turnover. Their action may also be dictated by whether they combine with ER-a or ER-b receptors.

Thyroid hormone receptors

Like other members of the nuclear receptor family, thyroid hormone receptors function as hormone-activated transcription factors. In contrast to steroid hormone receptors, however, thyroid hormone receptors bind to DNA in the absence of hormone, leading usually to transcriptional repression. When thyroid hormone binds to the receptor, however, it causes a conformational change in the receptor that changes it to function as a transcriptional activator. As with many other receptors, several isoforms have been discovered. Currently, four different isoforms are recognized, namely: α-1, α-2, β-1 and β-2. These different forms appear to be very important in development; different isoforms are expressed at different stages of development and in different organs and tissues. For example α-1, α-2 and βb-1 are expressed in virtually all tissues in which thyroid hormones act, but β-2 is synthesized mainly in the developing ear, and in the anterior pituitary gland and hypothalamus. Receptor α-1 is the first isoform detected in the conceptus, and the β form appears to be essential for normal brain development shortly after birth.

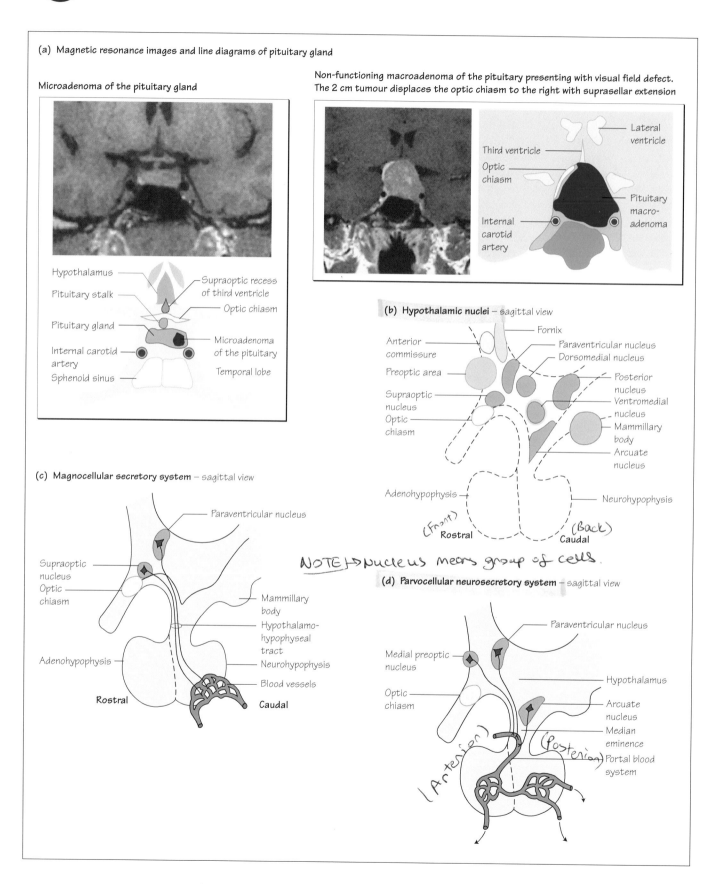

(a) Magnetic resonance images and line diagrams of pituitary gland

Microadenoma of the pituitary gland

Non-functioning macroadenoma of the pituitary presenting with visual field defect. The 2 cm tumour displaces the optic chiasm to the right with suprasellar extension

Lateral ventricle
Third ventricle
Optic chiasm
Internal carotid artery
Pituitary macro-adenoma

Hypothalamus
Pituitary stalk
Pituitary gland
Internal carotid artery
Sphenoid sinus
Supraoptic recess of third ventricle
Optic chiasm
Microadenoma of the pituitary
Temporal lobe

(b) Hypothalamic nuclei – sagittal view

Anterior commissure
Preoptic area
Supraoptic nucleus
Optic chiasm
Fornix
Paraventricular nucleus
Dorsomedial nucleus
Posterior nucleus
Ventromedial nucleus
Mammillary body
Arcuate nucleus
Adenohypophysis
Neurohypophysis
(Front) Rostral
(Back) Caudal

(c) Magnocellular secretory system – sagittal view

Paraventricular nucleus
Supraoptic nucleus
Optic chiasm
Mammillary body
Hypothalamo-hypophyseal tract
Neurohypophysis
Blood vessels
Adenohypophysis
Rostral
Caudal

NOTE→Nucleus means group of cells.

(d) Parvocellular neurosecretory system – sagittal view

Medial preoptic nucleus
Optic chiasm
Paraventricular nucleus
Hypothalamus
Arcuate nucleus
Median eminence
Portal blood system
(Arterior)
(Posterior)

Clinical scenario

A 51-year-old man was referred to the Endocrine Clinic as an emergency complaining of loss of vision in both sides of his visual field. He had been increasingly tired over the preceding few months, felt 'sluggish' and had lost all motivation for his usual activities. He was shaving less frequently than normal and had lost some body hair. He had also lost interest in sex, although put this down to his exhaustion and 'getting older'. More recently, he felt dizzy when he got out of bed or stood up from a chair. On examination he had clinical features of pan-hypopituitarism and examination of his visual fields revealed a bitemporal hemianopia. Biochemical investigations confirmed the presence of hyperprolactinaemia (serum prolactin 35 000 mU/L) and suppressed values of cortisol, thyroxine, TSH, LH, FSH, testosterone and IGF-1. An MRI scan showed a large pituitary tumour extending superiorly from the pituitary fossa and compressing the optic chiasm. He was treated with cabergoline, a long-acting dopamine agonist drug which subsequently caused shrinkage of the tumour. Examples of pituitary tumours are shown in Fig. 5a.

The hypothalamus

The hypothalamus lies at the base of the brain in the diencephalon. It contains a number of nuclei of neurones important in the regulation of hormone secretion from the pituitary. Some of these neurones produce hormones which are transported in the bloodstream to the pituitary. The hypothalamic boundaries are arbitrarily defined, in terms of visible structures around it, into the: rostral or supraoptic hypothalamus; middle or tuberal hypothalamus; and caudal or mamillary hypothalamus (Fig. 5b). Running longitudinally through the middle is the narrow **third ventricle**.

The medial hypothalamus contains a number of nuclei (Fig. 5b), densely packed with cells, which communicate with the rest of the brain through a bundle of descending and ascending axons: the **medial forebrain bundle**. The lateral zone of the hypothalamus does not have such well-defined nuclei. The **median eminence** of the hypothalamus is where the vascular link is made between the hypothalamic neurosecretory neurones and the pituitary gland.

The pituitary gland

The pituitary gland is distinguished as two main subglands, namely the anterior and posterior pituitary (Fig. 5b; adenohypophysis and neurohypophysis, respectively). Developmentally, the posterior gland is an outgrowth of the brain. During fetal development, it arises as a downward extrusion from the hypothalamus. It is thus neural in origin. The anterior pituitary grows upwards from the primitive oral cavity, which is termed Rathke's pouch. It grows upwards until it fuses with the downgrowing infundibulum, and its cells proliferate around and along the pituitary stalk, giving rise to the **pars tuberalis**. During development, a rich vascular system develops in the median eminence. The up-growth loses contact with the oral cavity, and the pituitary gland has direct neural contact with the hypothalamus, through to the posterior pituitary, and a vascular link, called the **portal system**, through which chemicals are carried from hypothalamic cells to the anterior pituitary gland.

Tumours of the pituitary may cause unrestrained hormone release, for example hyperprolactinaemia (see **Clinical scenario** and Fig. 5a).

The nuclei

Supraoptic group of nuclei: the paraventricular (PVN) and supraoptic (SON) nuclei have axons projecting to the posterior pituitary as the hypothalamic–hypophyseal tract. The PVN and SON contain large, richly vascularized cells, which together are termed the **magnocellular** secretory system (Fig. 5c). The PVN has other, smaller cells which contribute to a diffuse collection of hypothalamic neurones called the **parvocellular** secretory system (Fig. 5d), which, through the neurohormones it sends to the anterior pituitary, controls anterior pituitary function. Both the SON and PVN contain cells which produce and secrete important neuropeptides, for example oxytocin. The PVN is interconnected with autonomic and other regions of the spinal cord and the brain stem, as well as with the pituitary gland.

The tuberal or middle group of nuclei are involved in pituitary regulation. These are the ventromedial, dorsomedial and arcuate nuclei. Like the PVN, the ventromedial is interconnected with other parts of the brain, including the spinal cord, the brain stem and the central grey matter of the midbrain. The arcuate nucleus, which is an autonomous generator of reproductively important rhythms, sends many axons to the median eminence, as well as to other parts of the hypothalamus and forebrain.

The mammillary or posterior group of nuclei runs caudally into the mesencephalic central grey area. Within this area are more magnocellular neurones which project to many parts of the brain.

The neurohormones

The magnocellular neurones of the SON and the PVN contain neurones which produce and secrete **oxytocin** and **vasopressin** (antidiuretic hormone, ADH). The hormones are produced in different neurones and are transported to the posterior pituitary gland via their axons, which comprise the hypothalamic–hypophyseal tract.

The neurones of the parvocellular neurosecretory system send their axons to the median eminence, where their terminals release the 'releasing hormones': **corticotrophin-releasing hormone** (CRH); **gonadotrophin-releasing hormone** (GnRH); **thyrotrophin-releasing hormone** (TRH); and many other peptides, including somatostatin and neurotensin. Other substances emptied into the portal system include the dynorphins, enkephalins and β-endorphin, GABA, dopamine and many more substances.

GnRH neurones send axons not only to the median eminence, but to other parts of the brain, giving rise to the idea that GnRH may be a neurotransmitter as well as a prime regulator of fertility.

Cells of the PVN parvocellular system are rich in CRH and TRH, and project to the median eminence. The arcuate nucleus is rich in prolactin neurones, also called tubero-infundibular dopamine neurones. Arcuate neurones also contain the peptides galanin and growth hormone releasing hormone (GHRH), the opioids, somatostatin and several other substances, many of which are transported to the median eminence and the portal system.

6 Gonadotrophin-releasing hormone: a peptide hormone

(a) Synthesis and release of peptide hormones

1 Nucleus

DNA

| Initiation | Coding region |

Transcription

mRNA

2 Ribosomes

Translation

Cleavage

3 Endoplasmic reticulum

Preprohormone

Cleavage

Prohormone

4 Golgi apparatus

Cleavage

Hormone   Packaging
            Glycosylation

5 Granule

6 Secretion stimulus

Exocytosis

Secretion

(b) Gonadotrophin-releasing hormone (GnRH)

GnRH structure and function

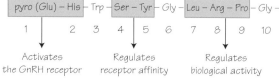

| pyro (Glu) – His | Trp | Ser – Tyr | Gly | Leu – Arg – Pro | Gly – |
| 1 | 2 | 3 | 4 | 5 | 6 | 7 | 8 | 9 | 10 |

Activates
the GnRH receptor

Regulates
receptor affinity

Regulates
biological activity

Table 6.1 Relative potency of some synthetic GnRH agonists

| Compound | Amino acid sequence | | | | | | | | | | Relative potency |
	1	2	3	4	5	6	7	8	9	10	
GnRH	pyroGlu	His	Trp	Ser	Tyr	Gly	Leu	Arg	Pro	Gly-NH$_2$	1
Leuprorelin	pyroGlu	His	Trp	Ser	Tyr	D-Leu	Leu	Arg	Pro	NCH$_3$CH$_2$NH$_2$	150
Deslorelin	pyroGlu	His	Trp	Ser	Tyr	D-Trp	Leu	Arg	Pro	NCH$_3$CH$_2$NH$_2$	1140

D- signifies the D-isomer of the amino acid

Clinical background

The therapeutic use of gonadotrophin-releasing hormone (GnRH) and its analogues is based on the discovery that pulsatile exposure of gonadotrophs to GnRH is required to maintain normal anterior pituitary function, whereas continuous GnRH secretion results in desensitization of the gonadotrophs and suppression of LH and FSH release. Thus GnRH or its analogues can be used in a pulsatile fashion to promote fertility in women with isolated GnRH deficiency or given continuously to suppress sex hormone secretion in patients with hormone-related cancers. Stable synthetic analogues of GnRH have been developed since GnRH, although used therapeutically as gonadorelin to assess pituitary function, is unstable and not satisfactory as a therapeutic agent. Stable analogues, including buserelin, goserelin, leuprorede, deslorelin and nafarelin, may be used to treat breast and prostate cancer, endometriosis, uterine fibroids and infertility.

Introduction

Gonadotrophin-releasing hormone (GnRH) is an excellent example of a peptide hormone for study, since so much is known about its chemistry, production, release and actions. GnRH is an hypothalamic peptide which is released in pulsatile fashion into the hypothalamo-hypophyseal portal blood system which supplies the anterior pituitary gland. This pulsatile secretion maintains the function of the anterior pituitary gonadotrophs in releasing the gonadotrophins LH and FSH which are necessary for proper ovarian and testicular function. This knowledge has led to the development of synthetic GnRH analogues.

Synthesis and release of peptide hormones

Transcription. The first step in the synthesis of a peptide such as GnRH is the transcription of the gene coding for the hormone mRNA (Fig. 6a). An initiation site on the gene, upstream from the coding region, is activated by a signal from the cytoplasm of the hypothalamic neurone in which it is synthesized. In the case of GnRH, the signal originates from a neurotransmitter, perhaps dopamine, which triggers an increase in cytoplasmic cAMP, resulting in activation of the gene. Conversely, cAMP production may be inhibited as a result of the action of an opioid neurotransmitter.

Preprohormone. The GnRH mRNA is called prepro-GnRH mRNA, since it will be translated into a large precursor peptide called prepro-GnRH. The mRNA moves out of the nucleus to the cytoplasm, where it is translated by ribosomes on the endoplasmic reticulum into prepro-GnRH. This precursor peptide consists of a signal sequence of 23 amino acids, followed by the sequence of GnRH itself and then by the 56 amino acids forming the C-terminal portion of the peptide. This latter portion is termed GAP (GnRH-associated peptide), which has been discovered to be an inhibitor of prolactin secretion. This highlights the principle that more than one physiologically active peptide can be generated from a single peptide precursor. The signal peptide directs its transfer to the endoplasmic reticulum, and during this processing it is cleaved to form a shorter prohormone.

Cleavage and packaging. From this point, the prohormone is transferred to the Golgi apparatus, where it is cleaved further to form the final hormone, in this case the decapeptide GnRH. The hormone is packaged into storage vesicles and released on demand, in this case as a cellular response to neurotransmitter activity.

Exocytosis. The hormone is released from the cell through the process of exocytosis. On stimulation, intracellular free Ca^{2+} and cAMP rise, causing contraction of myofilaments, and the vesicle is guided along microtubules to the cell membrane. The vesicle fuses with the membrane through a process which requires Ca^{2+}. The membrane is lysed and the contents are released into the extracellular space, and enter the bloodstream through neighbouring capillaries. GnRH neurone terminals impinge on the portal vessels, so that on release, a large proportion of exocytosed GnRH enters the portal system.

Structure-function studies

Once the structure of the hormone is elucidated, attempts are made to synthesize more stable analogues for therapeutic use, and, in the case of GnRH, substitution with D-amino acids produces potent analogues resistant to enzyme digestion (Fig. 6b; Table 6.1).

Receptor characterization. The stable analogues are radio-labelled and used to study the localization and properties of the peptide receptor. In the case of GnRH, these are situated on the plasma membrane of the anterior pituitary gonadotroph, and stimulation of the GnRH receptor by GnRH causes a rise in intracellular cAMP paralleled by the secretion of follicle-stimulating hormone (FSH) and luteinizing hormone (LH).

Hormone measurement. Once the hormone has been identified and synthesized in large quantities, antibodies can be raised against the hormone and used to measure it under different physiological and pathological conditions. In the case of GnRH, the availability of a radioimmunoassay enabled the discovery that the hormone is released episodically, approximately every 90 minutes. This episodic release is necessary to maintain gonadotrophin release, and thus fertility, in both the male and the female primate, including humans.

7 Principles of feedback control

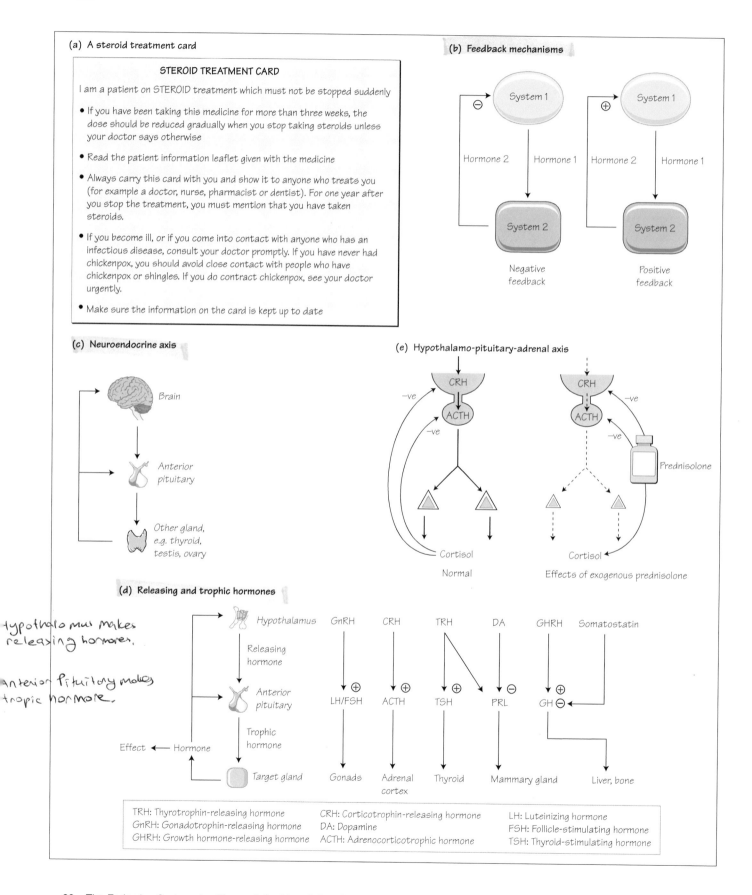

(a) A steroid treatment card

STEROID TREATMENT CARD

I am a patient on STEROID treatment which must not be stopped suddenly

- If you have been taking this medicine for more than three weeks, the dose should be reduced gradually when you stop taking steroids unless your doctor says otherwise

- Read the patient information leaflet given with the medicine

- Always carry this card with you and show it to anyone who treats you (for example a doctor, nurse, pharmacist or dentist). For one year after you stop the treatment, you must mention that you have taken steroids.

- If you become ill, or if you come into contact with anyone who has an infectious disease, consult your doctor promptly. If you have never had chickenpox, you should avoid close contact with people who have chickenpox or shingles. If you do contract chickenpox, see your doctor urgently.

- Make sure the information on the card is kept up to date

(b) Feedback mechanisms

Negative feedback

Positive feedback

(c) Neuroendocrine axis

Brain

Anterior pituitary

Other gland, e.g. thyroid, testis, ovary

(e) Hypothalamo-pituitary-adrenal axis

CRH

ACTH

Cortisol

Normal

CRH

ACTH

Prednisolone

Cortisol

Effects of exogenous prednisolone

(d) Releasing and trophic hormones

Hypothalamus

Releasing hormone

Anterior pituitary

Trophic hormone

Effect ← Hormone

Target gland

Hypothalamus makes releasing hormones.

Anterior Pituitary makes tropic hormone.

GnRH	CRH	TRH	DA	GHRH	Somatostatin
LH/FSH ⊕	ACTH ⊕	TSH ⊕	PRL ⊖	GH ⊕ ⊖	
Gonads	Adrenal cortex	Thyroid	Mammary gland	Liver, bone	

TRH: Thyrotrophin-releasing hormone
GnRH: Gonadotrophin-releasing hormone
GHRH: Growth hormone-releasing hormone

CRH: Corticotrophin-releasing hormone
DA: Dopamine
ACTH: Adrenocorticotrophic hormone

LH: Luteinizing hormone
FSH: Follicle-stimulating hormone
TSH: Thyroid-stimulating hormone

Clinical scenario

Glucocorticoid therapy is widely used to treat a variety of chronic inflammatory disorders. Mrs A.A. is a 69-year-old lady with long-standing rheumatoid arthritis. For the last 5 years she has taken oral prednisolone in a dose of 10 mg daily. She has developed some thinning of the skin and bruises easily, features which her doctor tells her are side-effects of the treatment. She knows that if she develops a minor illness she should increase the dose of her prednisolone for a couple of days and she carries a steroid card with her at all times (Fig. 7a). She also knows that if she starts vomiting for any reason she needs to seek urgent medical attention.

In the normal state, glucocorticoids are released in response to stress, such as illness. Therapeutic doses of glucocorticoids inhibit the normal hypothalamo–pituitary–adrenal feedback axis so that this stress response cannot occur. A patient such as Mrs A.A. relies entirely upon her fixed daily dose of prednisolone to supply her glucocorticoid requirements. If she develops a minor illness she needs to increase the dose of the tablets and if she is vomiting, needs to seek medical help so that glucocorticoids can be given intravenously. In the event that she stops taking glucocorticoids, she has to taper off the treatment gradually so as to allow the suppressed hypothalamo–pituitary–adrenal axis to recover normal function.

Homeostasis

Living systems possess their own internal environment, which has to survive within an external environment. Survival involves the maintenance of a fluid and salt balance, a tight control over temperature in the case of homoeotherms, and also over the regulation of chemical availability and utilization within the cell. Poikilotherms, for example some reptiles, whose temperature is set by the external environment, are more dependent on their external environment for maintenance of an adequate metabolism.

Internal control is achieved through integration of the different systems: neural, biochemical and physical. In all cases, the fundamental components of these systems are: (i) signals; (ii) transducers; (iii) sensors; and (iv) responders. The **signals** may be electrical impulses, or chemicals such as neurotransmitters, hormones or antigens. The **transducers** are poorly understood coupling systems which transform one form of energy into another, for example the conversion of an electrical impulse into a quantum of chemical neurotransmitter. **Sensors** are almost always receptors or enzymes or combined receptor–enzyme systems, which recognize specifically the signals which bind them. Transducers then convert the binding reaction into another electrical or chemical response. **Responders** are the apparatus of the cell that produce the final response, for example release or inhibition of hormone or neurotransmitter release, vasodilation, vasoconstriction or changes in heart rate.

Integration of endocrine systems is achieved through a complex interplay of regulatory feedback mechanisms operated through both hormonal and neural communication networks. The most important mechanisms are those commonly called **feedback**, whereby systems limit each other's activity around a preset oscillator.

For example system 1 (Fig. 7b) releases a hormone, hormone 1, which causes system 2, another gland, to release another hormone, hormone 2, which travels in the bloodstream. It is sensed by system 1, which somehow compares the concentration of the hormone with a comparator, and responds by altering the output of hormone 1. If system 1 responds by reducing the output of hormone 1, this is called a **negative-feedback** system. An example is the effect of thyroid hormone (hormone 2) from the thyroid gland (system 2), in reducing the output of thyroid-stimulating hormone (TSH; hormone 1) from the anterior pituitary gland (system 1; see Chapter 14).

If system 1 responds by increasing the output of hormone 1, this is called a **positive-feedback** system. An example is the effect of estrogen (hormone 2) from the ovary (system 2) on the release of luteinizing hormone (LH; hormone 1) from the anterior pituitary gland (system 1) just before ovulation (see Chapter 25).

In endocrinology, the brain–pituitary–target gland axes provide examples of feedback mechanisms in action (Fig. 7c). For virtually every anterior pituitary hormone, a corresponding hypothalamic releasing hormone has been discovered, and in some cases a corresponding inhibitory hypothalamic hormone has been found (Fig. 7d).

Feedback systems may involve more than two hormones, for example the control of thyroid hormone secretion. The brain releases thyrotrophin-releasing hormone, which travels down the portal blood system to the anterior pituitary thyrotroph cell, where it stimulates the release of TSH. TSH travels in the bloodstream to the thyroid gland, where it stimulates the release of T_3 and T_4. T_3 in turn inhibits TRH and TSH release. It will be readily apparent that this sort of system provides a means of testing the proper functioning of the feedback systems in health and disease.

One hypothalamic releasing hormone may release more than one anterior pituitary hormone. Gonadotrophin-releasing hormone (GnRH), releases both LH and FSH, which control gonadal steroidogenesis, ovarian follicular growth and ovulation in females and spermatogenesis in males.

Understanding basic feedback mechanisms is vital in clinical endocrinology where it forms the basis of diagnostic testing. For example the adrenal gland may develop a tumour which releases large amounts of cortisol. This feeds back to the brain and anterior pituitary gland suppressing the release of ACTH. In this case elevated serum cortisol levels in the presence of undetectable ACTH points to the adrenal as the source of the cortisol excess. If the diagnosis is a pituitary tumour secreting ACTH and therefore excess glucocorticoids, serum cortisol concentrations will be elevated in the presence of an inappropriately elevated ACTH concentration. Relatively large doses of glucocorticoids, for example prednisolone, prescribed for the patients with inflammatory or malignant diseases will also suppress the hypothalamo–pituitary–adrenal axis such that the patient switches off their endogenous cortisol production (see Clinical scenario; Fig. 7e). Ignorance of this feedback mechanism is potentially dangerous for the patient, whose stress response system is completely suppressed while on glucocorticoid therapy. This must be withdrawn gradually to allow the system to restore normal cortisol secretion.

8 Endocrine function tests

(a) Principles of endocrine function testing

Most hormones:
- Are subject to diurnal or ultradian rhythms
- Are secreted in a pulsatile fashion
- Are controlled by feedback from target organs (usually negative)
- Develop autonomous secretion in pathological states

As a general rule:
- If the clinical suspicion is of hormone excess then suppression tests are used
- If the clinical suspicion is of hormone deficiency then stimulation tests are used

The chemical pathology laboratory must ensure that assays are:
- Sensitive
- Specific
- Reproducible
- Subject to internal and external quality control

(c) Sample record of an ITT

PATIENT DETAILS				CONSULTANT		
Name, dob, hospital number etc				Dr I.N.Charge		

DIAGNOSIS AND REASON FOR TEST
Exclude hypopituitarism

TESTS REQUESTED
ITT please

NOTES			
ECG – normal	Basal cortisol – 270nmol/L	H/O Epilepsy – No	Weight – 70kg

PRESCRIPTION		SIGNATURE	DATE
Actrapid 0.15 Units/kg = 10.5 units IV x 1 dose		D.R. Oncall	22.12.10

Time	Time taken	Treatment / comments	Glucometer	Lab glucose	Cortisol	GH
-15	0845		4.0	3.9	290	0.7
0	0900	Insulin 10.5 units IV				
+15	0915		2.9	2.9	275	8.0
+25	0925	Sweaty, tachycardia	2.1	2.0	300	35
+30	0930	Feels nauseated, sweaty	1.9	1.7	290	40
+45	0945		3.0	3.0	560	44
+60	1000		3.4	3.3	600	60
+75	1015	Feeling better	3.5	3.5	650	25
+90	1030		3.9	3.8	610	14
+120	1100	Fine. Given sandwiches at end of test	3.9	4.0	600	3.5

(b) Examples of dynamic endocrine function tests and their uses

Test	Type	Uses	Comments
Insulin Tolerance Test (ITT)	Stimulation	Diagnosis of ACTH deficiency Diagnosis of GH Deficiency	Contraindicated in patients with significant ischaemic heart disease, epilepsy, glycogen storage diseases or severe hypoadrenalism. May combine with GnRH and TRH in "Combined Pituitary Function Test" – see Chapter 5
Glucagon test	Stimulation	Diagnosis of hypopituitarism Diagnosis of GH Deficiency	Tests the hypothalamic–pituitary axis when ITT contraindicated
Oral Glucose Tolerance Test (OGTT)	Suppression	Diagnosis of acromegaly	GH fails to suppress normally in acromegaly – see Chapter 12
Oral Glucose Tolerance Test (OGTT)	Stimulation	Diagnosis of diabetes mellitus	Exaggerated glucose response in diabetes – see Chapter 41
Midnight/0900h cortisols	Basal/diurnal	Confirm suspicion of Cushing's Syndrome	Loss of diurnal rhythm in Cushing's syndrome. Midnight sample: patient must be asleep
Overnight, low- and high-dose dexamethasone suppression tests	Suppression	Diagnosis of Cushing's syndrome	In normal subjects, cortisol undetectable at 0900h following low dose of dexamethasone the previous midnight. Low- and high- dose suppression tests may distinguish between pituitary, adrenal and ectopic cortisol excess – see Chapter 17
Short Synacthen Test (SST)	Stimulation	Diagnosis of primary adrenal failure (Addison's Disease)	Failure of rise in cortisol secretion after synthetic ACTH (Synacthen) indicates adrenal failure – see Chapter 21

 The Endocrine System at a Glance, 3rd edition. © Ben Greenstein and Diana Wood. Published 2011 by Blackwell Publishing Ltd.

Clinical setting

In general, patients with endocrine disorders present to clinicians because they are thought to have either hormone excess or hormone deficiency and each of these states has a variety of underlying causes. The accurate diagnosis of clinical endocrine disease depends upon knowledge of the principles of feedback control described in Chapter 7, on an understanding of basic endocrine biochemistry and on the availability of high quality assay systems provided by chemical pathology laboratories (Fig. 8a).

Many hormones are secreted in a pulsatile fashion, often subject to diurnal or ultradian rhythms, such that a single, untimed blood sample may be of little or no diagnostic value. There are important exceptions to this rule, in particular thyroid disease in which basal measurements of TSH and free thyroid hormone concentrations are diagnostic in the vast majority of cases, hyperprolactinaemia in which a single result in an unstressed patient is reliable and calcium and PTH measurements which are stable. Characteristically, endocrine disorders disrupt normal feedback mechanisms and this feature is exploited in the interpretation of a number of endocrine function tests. Furthermore, certain hormones rise in response to stressful stimuli and this too can be utilized for diagnostic purposes. Because of these special considerations, collection of anything other than basal and straightforward blood samples must be undertaken by experienced staff who are aware of the appropriate local protocols. In hospital endocrine referral centres, specialist nurses are skilled in correct patient preparation for the tests, the delivery of drugs required for hormone stimulation or suppression, careful clinical monitoring of patients, observation for side effects during the tests and correct management of samples. The latter forms a vital part of dynamic testing protocols and more complex investigations should always be performed in conjunction with chemical pathology staff to ensure that samples are collected into the correct preservatives at the necessary temperature and maintained in ideal conditions prior to transfer to the laboratory.

Careful recording of the timing of the test, any symptoms experienced by the patient and the results are essential.

There are many dynamic function tests employed in clinical endocrinology and clinicians must refer to local protocols and normal ranges. Examples of some commonly used dynamic endocrine function tests are shown in Fig. 8b. Two examples follow which illustrate some important principles of endocrine testing.

Insulin tolerance test

The insulin tolerance test (ITT) is used to assess the anterior pituitary reserve of growth hormone (GH) and adrenocorticotrophin (ACTH), both of which are stress hormones and rise in response to illness and hypoglycaemia. The ITT tests the response to a hypoglycaemic stimulus which acts at the level of the hypothalamus to stimulate the production of these pituitary counter-regulatory hormones. The ITT is contraindicated in patients with significant ischaemic heart disease, epilepsy, glycogen storage diseases and severe hypoadrenalism (0900h cortisol <100 nmol/l). Thus a 0900h cortisol measurement and ECG must be performed prior to the test and 25% dextrose and hydrocortisone available for intravenous injection during the test if required. An experienced nurse and a doctor must be present throughout and resuscitation equipment be available. If in doubt, a glucagon test should replace the ITT, although it produces less reliable results.

Patients fast from 2200h the night before the test, which should start at 0900h. After weighing, soluble insulin (Actrapid) is given as a bolus dose of 0.15 U/kg. Blood samples are taken for glucose, cortisol and GH at regular intervals – the blood glucose must fall below 2.2 mmol/l to provide an adequate hypoglycaemic stimulus (further insulin may be given if this is not achieved). At the end of the test the patient must be given food to eat and 100 mg iv hydrocortisone if the hypoglycaemia was severe. Fig. 8c shows a typical ITT recording chart. Results may vary from laboratory to laboratory and advice about normal responses should be checked locally. In general, severe GH deficiency is indicated by a peak GH of 3 μg/L or less and a normal peak cortisol should exceed 550 nmol/L.

Water deprivation test

A water deprivation test (WDT) is performed when there is a clinical suspicion of either central or nephrogenic diabetes insipidus (see Chapter 36) or to investigate thirst and polyuria. Like the ITT, extreme care is needed to perform a WDT and constant supervision to prevent the patient from drinking, to monitor body weight and to handle plasma and urine samples appropriately. Extreme caution should be taken in patients with severe DI and the diagnosis may be made on overnight basal samples alone where the plasma osmolality is >295 mosmol/kg and the urine osmolality/plasma osmolality ratio (U/P) is <2.0.

Before starting the WDT the patient should be allowed to drink freely to 0800h but should avoid tea, coffee or smoking. The patient should be weighed and 97% of this weight recorded. From 0800h all fluid intake is discontinued for 8 hours. The patient is weighed and urine and plasma samples taken hourly for measurement of urine volume and urine and plasma osmolalities. If the weight loss exceeds 3% of body weight the test is discontinued, plasma osmolality measured urgently and desmopressin given if osmolality >305 mosmol/kg. Assuming the test continues, at 1600h desmopressin 2 μg is given intramuscularly and urine and plasma samples continued for a further 4h.

In cranial diabetes insipidus the plasma osmolality rises with inappropriately high urine volumes and no evidence of concentration. After desmopressin, urine volumes fall with normal concentration. In nephrogenic diabetes insipidus the urine fails to concentrate after desmopressin injection. Results in primary polydipsia are variable and urine concentration may not maximize due to previous high urine volumes causing a decrease in the osmotic gradient in the loop of Henle.

9 Growth: I Cellular growth factors

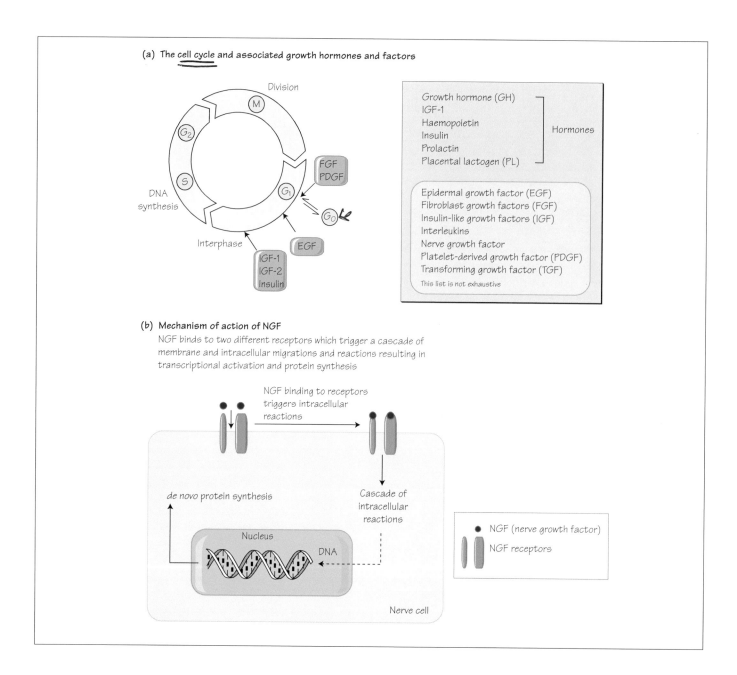

(a) The cell cycle and associated growth hormones and factors

Division

M

G₂

S

DNA synthesis

Interphase

G₁

FGF
PDGF

G₀

EGF

IGF-1
IGF-2
Insulin

Growth hormone (GH)
IGF-1
Haemopoietin
Insulin
Prolactin
Placental lactogen (PL)

Hormones

Epidermal growth factor (EGF)
Fibroblast growth factors (FGF)
Insulin-like growth factors (IGF)
Interleukins
Nerve growth factor
Platelet-derived growth factor (PDGF)
Transforming growth factor (TGF)

This list is not exhaustive

(b) Mechanism of action of NGF

NGF binds to two different receptors which trigger a cascade of membrane and intracellular migrations and reactions resulting in transcriptional activation and protein synthesis

NGF binding to receptors triggers intracellular reactions

de novo protein synthesis

Cascade of intracellular reactions

Nucleus

DNA

NGF (nerve growth factor)

NGF receptors

Nerve cell

Clinical background

Tumours secreting IGF-1 and IGF-2 have been described in humans. They are very rare! The tumours are part of the group of neuroendocrine tumours, the most common of which are carcinoids. Patients with neuroendocrine tumours may present with severe hypoglycaemic episodes and confirmed hypoglycaemia in non-diabetic patients should always be investigated. The primary tumour may be difficult to localize and the patient requires specialist treatment from a multidisciplinary team of endocrinologists, surgeons, radiologists and oncologists.

Cellular growth and proliferation
The cell cycle

The growth phase is G_1, which prepares the cell for the synthetic phase S, during which the DNA becomes duplicated (Fig. 9a). The cell splits into two daughter cells in the M phase. The new cells may thereafter remain in G_0 (e.g. neurones, muscle cells), or enter G_1 to repeat the cycle. Tumour cells may remain in G_0, before re-entering G_1. Growth factors and hormones act at specific phases of the cell cycle.

 The Endocrine System at a Glance, 3rd edition. © Ben Greenstein and Diana Wood. Published 2011 by Blackwell Publishing Ltd.

Growth factors

Insulin-like growth factors (IGF-1, IGF-2). IGF-1 and IGF-2 mediate the actions of growth hormone and have other important metabolic effects. GH causes the release of IGF-1 and IGF-2 from the liver, although IGF-1 is the most GH dependent. Both circulate in plasma bound to proteins known as IGF-binding proteins (IGF-BPs), of which six specific types have been described. Cellular responses to IGF are mediated by specific IGF receptors, which are similar to but distinct from insulin receptors. Plasma levels of IGF-1 and IGF-2 remain fairly constant in the healthy adult due to the stability of their binding proteins. IGF-1 mRNA can be detected in numerous body tissues and is thought to play a GH-independent role in tissue growth. Its production is stimulated by insulin and the hyperinsulinaemia of obesity may affect circulating IGF-1 and IGF-BP concentrations.

Insulin. Apart from its role in the control of carbohydrate metabolism, insulin is an anabolic hormone. Without insulin, protein catabolism is enhanced and amino acid uptake into muscle is inhibited, as is the translation of mRNA.

Placental lactogen (PL) is a placental hormone. Many of the actions of PL are similar to those of prolactin. PL promotes growth of the mammary duct system, milk protein synthesis and the incorporation of sulphur into cartilage. PL may play a role in mammary gland development and in preparation for the action of prolactin after parturition. PL antagonizes the actions of insulin, and promotes amino acid and glucose utilization in the fetus. During the second trimester of pregnancy, PL may take over the role of chorionic gonadotrophin, the levels of which begin to decline.

Prolactin (PRL) promotes milk synthesis. Together with adrenal steroids and estrogens, PRL stimulates mammary duct system growth.

Nerve growth factor (NGF) is similar in structure to proinsulin. It is secreted in large amounts by the submandibular glands, under the control of tri-iodothyronine, thyroxine and testosterone, and is therefore present in much larger quantities in the saliva of the male. NGF is critically important in nerve growth and regeneration and may play a role in fighting, since it is released into the bloodstream in huge amounts when male mice fight each other. NGF, in common with most other growth factors, binds to membrane receptors to trigger an intracellular cascade of reactions resulting in *de novo* protein synthesis (Fig. 9b).

Injection of NGF antiserum into the developing rat embryo causes widespread damage to the sympathetic division of the autonomic nervous system. NGF induces neurite growth and plays a role in the guidance of growing sympathetic fibres to the organs they will ultimately innervate. Cells in the path of the growing axon synthesize and release NGF. In the brain, NGF may have a role in maintaining memory, since it restores learning and memory to rats with brain lesions, which suggests that NGF may be useful in Alzheimer's disease.

Epidermal growth factor (EGF) is a 53 amino acid peptide, isolated from the mouse salivary gland, where it is associated with an EGF-binding protein. EGF is released by α-adrenergic agonists, suggesting that release is under autonomic control. In the embryo and neonatal mouse, EGF promotes proliferation of the cells of the epidermis, the opening of the eyelids and the eruption of teeth. EGF promotes the maturation of the epithelium of developing lungs, keratinization of the skin and phosphorylation of proteins. EGF is present in breast milk as a mitogenic factor.

Transforming growth factors (TGF). TGF-α and TGF-β are peptides which cause the growth of fibroblast cells. TGF-α is a 50 amino acid peptide, structurally similar to EGF. It binds to the EGF receptor and shares many of the actions of EGF. TGF-α itself exists in at least five forms (TGF-α-1 to TGF-α-5).

TGF-β also exists in at least five forms (TGF-β-1 to TGF-β-5) and was originally discovered in platelets. It is present in most cells, especially in bone matrix where it may be important in chondrocyte, osteoblast and osteoclast differentiation and growth.

TGF-β can be stimulatory or inhibitory to the growth of non-endothelial cells, depending on the presence or absence of other factors. It does not bind to the EGF receptor. It may be inhibitory or stimulatory to organ and tumour growth, and modulates the action of other growth factors, including that of EGF. TGF-β has structural homology with the Müllerian inhibiting hormone and inhibin.

The fibroblast growth factor (FGF) family includes acidic, basic, keratinocyte and other polypeptide growth factors which share several properties, including substantial sequence homology, angiogenesis promotion, heparin binding and mitogenic action in several different cell types. They are also called heparin-binding growth factors (HBGF). Binding to heparin stabilizes the factors and enhances their biological activities.

Platelet-derived growth factor (PDGF) is synthesized and stored in blood platelets, and released when platelets are activated during blood vessel injury. Other tissues synthesize and store PDGF. The peptide is a heterodimer consisting of A and B chains, and forms part of a larger family consisting of PDGF (AA), (AB) and (BB). AB is the predominant form present in platelets. There are two different receptors for PDGF, one which recognizes all the heterodimers, and one which recognizes only BB. PDGF is a powerful cell growth promoter *in vitro*, has strong chemotactic properties and appears to have a role in inflammation and tumour and cell growth.

Erythropoietin is erythrocyte-stimulating factor, produced in the kidneys, which travels to the bone marrow to stimulate production of mature red blood cells. In plasma, erythropoietin has a half-life of 5 hours, while its effects are not manifested for at least 36 hours, a time sequence consistent with the probability that erythropoietin generates a sequence of haemopoietic events which are not dependent on its continuous presence for completion.

The interleukins are a family of at least eight proteins. They are examples of the cytokines, a group of soluble proteins which act as intercellular communicators. IL-1 is produced by activated macrophages, and stimulates IL-2 production by T cells and proliferation and differentiation of B cells. IL-2 is produced by T cells activated during an immune response. IL-6 is interferon-β, which is synthesized by fibroblasts and some tumour cells. It increases immunoglobulin synthesis, and has antiviral activity.

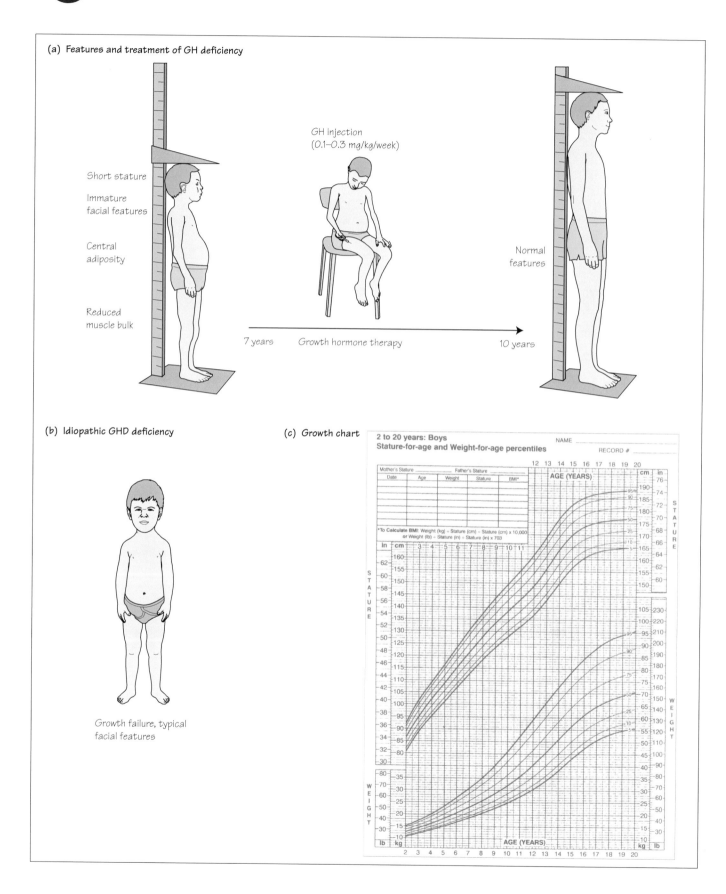

(a) Features and treatment of GH deficiency

Short stature

Immature facial features

Central adiposity

Reduced muscle bulk

GH injection (0.1–0.3 mg/kg/week)

7 years   Growth hormone therapy   10 years

Normal features

(b) Idiopathic GHD deficiency

Growth failure, typical facial features

(c) Growth chart

2 to 20 years: Boys
Stature-for-age and Weight-for-age percentiles

Clinical background

Short stature in children is a common presenting complaint. The majority of short children do not have an identifiable abnormality and thus it is important to make accurate measurements of height over a period of time and to calculate growth velocity. Short stature can reflect a wide range of underlying causes, ranging from nutritional and psychosocial factors, to endocrine disorders and genetic dysmorphic syndromes.

Growth hormone deficiency (GHD; Fig. 10a) has numerous causes related to congenital midline structural defects of the hypothalamus and pituitary, acquired lesions following perinatal trauma or central nervous system infections, primary and secondary tumours of the hypothalamus and pituitary, autoimmune hypophysitis and following cranial irradiation. In the majority of cases the cause is unknown ('idiopathic' GHD; Fig. 10b). Children with GHD present with growth failure and typical features relating to GH effects on bone and body composition. Thus the facial appearance is immature with a depressed central zone and prominent forehead related to lack of GH effects on skull maturation. GHD children have reduced muscle bulk and increased central fat deposition consistent with a lack of the metabolic effects of GH. Untreated they will reach approximately 65 to 70% of predicted adult height and this can be reversed by the introduction of GH replacement therapy at the earliest possible age (Fig. 10a).

Normal growth
Prenatal growth

The growth rate is an informative index of mental and physical development, both pre- and postnatally. Normal intrauterine growth and development are critically dependent on maternal diet and state of health and adversely affected by excessive maternal alcohol intake and smoking. Endocrine influences on intrauterine growth and development are poorly understood.

Circulating maternal **unconjugated estriol** is an important index of normal fetal growth. Estriol's function is not understood but it is known to be produced by the placenta using precursor steroids derived from both fetus and mother. Table 10.1 shows expected ranges during pregnancy. Reduced values may point to the possibility of intrauterine growth retardation or Down's syndrome (Table 10.2).

Postnatal growth

Human postnatal growth in stature and weight is assessed relative to standardized growth curves (Fig. 10c). Growth rates are highest during fetal development and just after birth. There is a spurt in growth in boys and girls between 6½ and 7 years, followed by a plateau and then the sharp pubertal growth spurt. Growth ceases with the fusion of the long bone epiphyses by sex steroids, reflecting full adult growth and maturation.

Normal growth is influenced by genetic, socioeconomic and nutritional factors, and chronic disease. There is a good correlation between parental and child height which is sex-specific. The correlations with respect to birth length, rate of growth and final height are well documented in families. Poor hygiene, poverty and malnutrition adversely affect growth before and after parturition. Smoking, alcohol and drug abuse have deleterious effects on the fetus and growing child. Malnutrition is associated with several adverse effects on the endocrine system, including decreased concentrations of circulating IGF-1, decreased GH receptors and post-GH receptor defects with the predicted elevation of serum GH.

Any form of chronic disease, particularly when associated with malabsorption, such as coeliac disease or inflammatory bowel disease, may impair growth and should be excluded before subjecting a child to lengthy endocrine investigation of short stature.

Endocrine hormones are essential for postnatal growth. Growth hormone (GH) exerts its effects directly and through the mediation of the insulin-like growth factors. Disorders of GH synthesis, secretion or action may originate in the hypothalamus, pituitary gland, at sites of IGF-1 production or at target organs for the hormones. Thus GH abnormalities in children may present with low or absent circulating GH concentrations (as in idiopathic GH deficiency) or with the elevated GH levels seen in association with GH receptor abnormalities in the Laron syndrome.

Thyroid hormones are essential for normal intrauterine and postnatal development; fetal thyroid deficiencies cause mental impairment and delayed development, but whilst postnatally acquired hypothyroidism inhibits growth it does not usually affect mental development. Excess glucocorticoid treatment in childhood can also impair growth. The gonadal sex steroids are essential for the normal pubertal growth spurt and individuals with delayed puberty present with short stature as well as developmental delay.

Table 10.1 Expected ranges of estriol levels in pregnancy

Weeks of gestation	Expected range (ng/mL)	Weeks of gestation	Expected range (ng/mL)	Twin pregnancy (ng/mL)
12	0.3–1.0	22–23	2.7–16	3–18
13	0.3–1.1	24–25	2.9–17	3–20
14	0.4–1.6	26–27	3.0–18	4–21
15	1.0–4.4	28–29	3.2–20	4–22
16	1.4–6.5	30–31	3.6–22	5–25
17	1.5–6.6	32–33	4.6–23	6–39
18	1.6–8.5	34–35	5.1–25	7–39
19	1.9–11	36–37	7.2–29	9–38
20	2.1–13	38–39	7.8–37	13–40
21	2.6–14	40–42	8.0–39	–

Table 10.2 Estriol levels in pregnancy (Down's syndrome)

Weeks of gestation[a]	N	Median (nmol/L)	Median (ng/mL)
15	19	5.34	1.54
16	108	7.11	2.05
17	371	8.91	2.57
18	162	10.68	3.08
19	74	12.45	3.59
20	22	14.25	4.11
21	16	16.01	4.62

[a] 15th week of gestation means 14 weeks + x days (x < 7); values taken by ultrasound scan. N: number of observations.

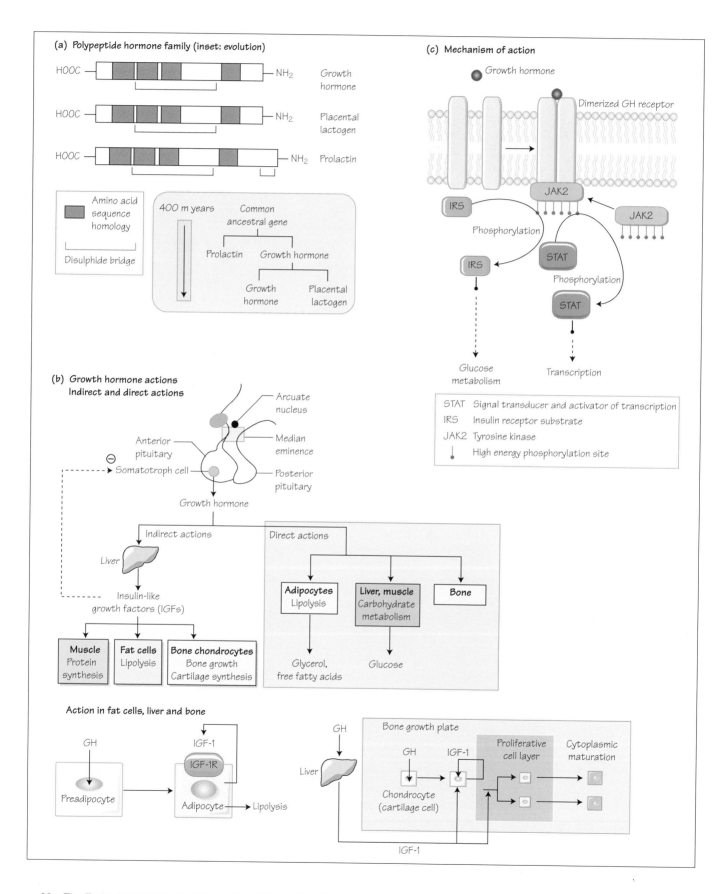

(a) Polypeptide hormone family (inset: evolution)

(b) Growth hormone actions
Indirect and direct actions

Action in fat cells, liver and bone

(c) Mechanism of action

STAT   Signal transducer and activator of transcription
IRS   Insulin receptor substrate
JAK2   Tyrosine kinase
       High energy phosphorylation site

Clinical background

Growth hormone is necessary for the maintenance of good health in adult life as well as for the promotion of growth in childhood. Adults with growth hormone deficiency (GHD) are physically and psychologically less well than normal subjects due to the diverse nature of GH action. The vast majority of patients with adult GHD have pre-existing hypothalamic–pituitary disease, generally a pituitary adenoma. GHD may be part of the presenting illness or may be induced by pituitary surgery or radiotherapy used in treatment. A small percentage of patients with adult GHD will have presented with idiopathic GHD in childhood.

The adult GHD syndrome is characterized by abnormalities of metabolism, body composition and bone density and by psychological features of low mood, poor self-esteem, anxiety and social isolation. Adults with GHD have increased risk factors for cardiac disease reflected in reduced lean body mass, increased central fat deposition, raised cholesterol and harmful low-density lipoprotein concentrations and evidence of increased atheromatous deposits throughout the arterial system. Bone mineral density is reduced and there is an increased risk of fractures. The poor quality of life is a striking feature of the syndrome and has been demonstrated using recognized assessments of psychological health. GH replacement therapy is given as a daily subcutaneous injection of recombinant human GH.

Growth hormone (GH)
Chemistry and synthesis

GH is synthesized in the somatotroph cells in the anterior pituitary gland. GH is a member of a family of polypeptide hormones, including prolactin (PRL) and placental lactogen (PL; Fig. 11a). GH is a single chain 191 amino acid polypeptide, and has a high structural homology with PL and PRL. All three are derived from a common precursor, even though each hormone has its own gene. They share a common ancestral gene from which the GH/PL gene diverged about 400 million years ago, and divergence of GH and PL genes occurred about 85 to 100 million years ago. The GH and PL genes exist as multiple copies on chromosome 17, and the PRL gene is a single copy on chromosome 6. Mouse fibroblasts synthesize a peptide called proliferin, which has significant structural homology with GH, PRL and PL, suggesting that this family may be larger than originally appreciated. GH and PRL exist in pituitary and plasma in more than one form, that is they show structural heterogeneity.

Actions of growth hormone (Fig. 11b)

The most dramatic action of GH is on muscle and skeletal bone growth. The actions may be conveniently divided into direct and indirect actions.

Indirect actions of growth hormone. GH acts in the liver to stimulate the synthesis and secretion of the peptide IGF-1 which stimulates bone growth. In **fat cells**, IGF-1 stimulates lipolysis and in **muscle**, it stimulates protein synthesis. Functional GH receptors also exist in bone, stimulating local production of IGF-1 in proliferative chondrocytes.

The direct actions of GH have been termed diabetogenic, since the hormone's actions oppose those of insulin, being lipolytic in fat and gluconeogenic in muscle. These actions are implicated in disorders of GH action.

Growth hormone receptor (Fig. 11c). The mechanism of action of GH is still under investigation. It has a specific receptor on the membrane of the target cell. The growth hormone receptor is a polypeptide of 619 residues which is organized into three distinct domains, viz. an extracellular ligand binding domain, a single transmembrane segment and an intracellular domain. It is part of the haematopoietic type I cytokine receptor family. The extracellular domain of the GH receptor consists of 192 residues and has been found on the receptor and as a circulating isoform protein called growth hormone receptor binding protein, which is used as a marker of receptor number integrity. It appears that each asymmetrical molecule of GH binds two homologous binding domains on two separate GH receptors, and that there is a sequential effect, in that one part of the GH molecule must bind first to its site on one receptor followed by the other binding reaction to another receptor, for the cell to respond appropriately.

Signal transduction. No changes in cAMP or phosphoinositol (the PLC/IP3 systems) have been reported. After the binding reactions have occurred, the cytoplasmic domain of the receptor recruits the tyrosine kinase JAK2, and phosphorylation of the receptor and the JAK2 occurs. Phosphotyrosine residues on both JAK2 and the growth hormone receptor have docking sites for several intracellular signalling proteins which possess phosphotyrosine motifs, for example SH2 domains. Thus, the growth hormone–receptor complex somehow enables JAK2 to phosphorylate a number of different proteins, resulting in the cellular response. The substrates for phosphorylation by JAK2 include the insulin receptor substrate (IRS), the glucocorticoid receptor, the epidermal growth factor receptor, signal transducers and activators of transcription (STATS) and several others.

The cellular response depends on which of these molecules becomes phosphorylated, and the result may be, for example, a metabolic change or transcriptional activation or repression. For example activation of the insulin receptor substrate results in the insulin-like actions of growth hormone, while activation of STAT causes transcriptional activation. The growth hormone receptor is regulated by inhibitory intracellular proteins which prevent unregulated growth. Examples of regulators include: (i) SH2-domain-containing protein tyrosine phosphatases which dephosphorylate the receptor and the JAK2 tyrosine kinase; and (ii) suppressors of cytokine signalling (SOCS), which bind to JAK2 and block its kinase activity. These basic research discoveries are of great interest as possible new approaches to the treatment of growth hormone-related diseases.

(a) Clinical features of acromegaly

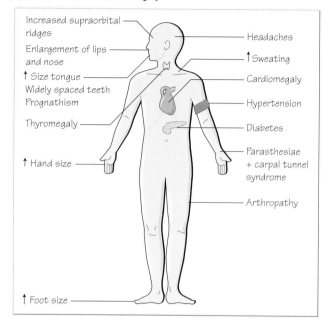

Increased supraorbital ridges
Enlargement of lips and nose
↑ Size tongue
Widely spaced teeth
Prognathism
Thyromegaly
↑ Hand size
↑ Foot size

Headaches
↑ Sweating
Cardiomegaly
Hypertension
Diabetes
Parasthesiae + carpal tunnel syndrome
Arthropathy

(c) Hands in acromegaly compared with normal hand (middle)

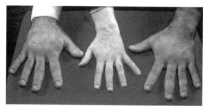

(d) Widely spaced dentition in a patient with acromegaly

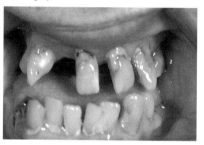

(e) The facial appearance of a man with acromegaly

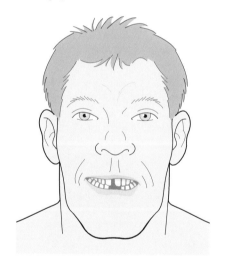

(b) Regulation of growth hormone secretion

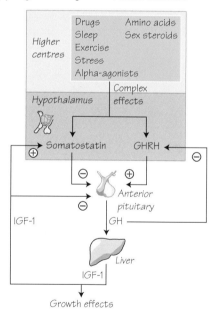

Higher centres
Drugs   Amino acids
Sleep   Sex steroids
Exercise
Stress
Alpha-agonists

Complex effects
Hypothalamus
⊕ Somatostatin   GHRH ⊖
⊖   ⊕
Anterior pituitary
⊖
IGF-1   GH
Liver
IGF-1
Growth effects

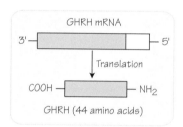

GHRH mRNA
3'   5'
Translation
COOH   NH₂
GHRH (44 amino acids)

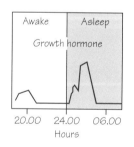

Awake   Asleep
Growth hormone
20.00   24.00   06.00
Hours

30 *The Endocrine System at a Glance*, 3rd edition. © Ben Greenstein and Diana Wood. Published 2011 by Blackwell Publishing Ltd.

Clinical scenario

Excess growth hormone (GH) secretion causes the typical syndrome of acromegaly. Mr SJ was a 53-year-old chef who had generally been well and rarely went to the doctor. On this occasion he presented to his GP because of aches and pains in the joints of his hands which were causing a problem with his work. The GP thought he looked acromegalic and asked him a series of questions related to his symptoms, following which he established a number of abnormalities on examination. He referred Mr SJ to the local Endocrine Clinic where biochemical investigations confirmed the diagnosis of acromegaly. In particular, his plasma GH level was elevated at 25 mcg/L and failed to suppress during a glucose tolerance test and his plasma IGF-1 concentration was five times the upper limit of normal. An MRI scan of the pituitary revealed a pituitary macroadenoma rising out of the pituitary fossa into the suprasellar space but not compressing the optic chiasm. He had a good response to pituitary surgery and subsequent radiotherapy, with resolution of many of the features of acromegaly. The clinical features of acromegaly are shown in Fig. 12a.

Regulation of growth hormone secretion

Growth hormone (GH) secretion is regulated primarily by the hypothalamus, which produces growth hormone-releasing hormone (GHRH; Fig. 12b). This action is integrated with the action of a hormone called **ghrelin**, secreted mainly by epithelial cells lining the fundus of the stomach. Ghrelin is a potent releaser of GH from the anterior pituitary gland by binding to pituitary GH receptors, and is also involved in energy balance (see Chapter 45).

GHRH in humans is a 44 amino acid peptide, which is released into the portal system and binds to specific receptors on anterior pituitary somatotrophs to stimulate GH release. The second messenger activated by GHRH is cAMP, although the IP3 system may also be activated. The hypothalamus also produces an inhibitory hormone called **somatostatin**, which inhibits GH release from somatotrophs. Somatostatin is a 14 amino acid peptide, which also exists in the hypothalamus in a 28 amino acid form. Both are active in inhibiting GH secretion, which they do by inhibiting cAMP production. Both GHRH and somatostatin have been localized to the arcuate nucleus (see Chapter 5). GH is released in a pulsatile fashion with the major peak in secretion occurring about one hour after the onset of sleep. In adults, circulating GH levels are low or undetectable for most of the day with intermittent bursts of secretion being observed. Somatostatinergic tone is felt to be the most important determinant of production of a GH peak – troughs in somatostatin production being associated with a GHRH peak and subsequent GH release. The physiological feedback control of GH release is mediated by insulin-like growth factor (IGF-1), which stimulates somatostatin secretion from the hypothalamus and inhibits GH secretion directly.

Pathophysiology of growth hormone secretion
GH deficiency

Causes of GH deficiency are either genetic, resulting in short stature in children (Chapter 10) or acquired, leading to the adult GHD syndrome. GH deficiency is treated by replacement with human growth hormone (hGH). Originally extracted from post-mortem human pituitaries, nowadays hGH is synthesized using recombinant DNA techniques, which obviates the hazards inherent in using human-derived material, which carries with it the danger of infection.

GH excess

Excess secretion of GH results in **acromegaly** in adults (see Clinical scenario) and **gigantism** in young adults if affected before fusion of the bony epiphyses. The usual source of excess GH secretion is a pituitary adenoma. Rarely, ectopic neuroendocrine tumours secreting GHRH occur, either in isolation or as part of the MEN 1 syndrome (Chapter 50). Acromegaly results in a coarsening of the facial features and of the soft tissues of the hands (Fig. 12c) and feet. Exaggerated growth of the mandible (lower jaw) occurs, resulting in a characteristic facial configuration (Fig. 12d and e). There is hypertrophy of connective tissue of the kidney, heart and liver, and the patient's glucose tolerance is lowered by up to 50%, resulting in diabetes in about 10% of patients with acromegaly. Other symptoms include headaches, sweating, renal colic due to nephrolithiasis and arthralgia. A diagnosis of acromegaly is confirmed by the failure of elevated GH levels to suppress during an oral glucose tolerance test, coupled with elevated serum IGF-1 concentrations.

The treatment of choice for acromegaly is surgical removal of the pituitary adenoma, plus or minus adjunctive radiotherapy or medical treatment with somatostatin analogues or dopamine agonists. Untreated, acromegaly is associated with increased mortality from cardiovascular disease and cancer.

13 Thyroid: I Thyroid gland and thyroid hormones

(a) Patient with a large multinodular goitre

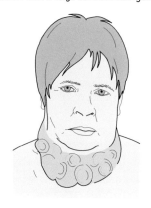

(b) Position of thyroid in neck

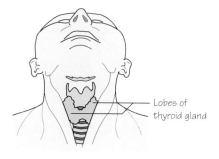

Lobes of thyroid gland

(c) Thyroid-hormone synthesis

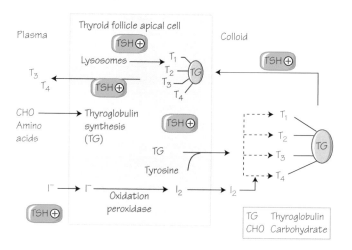

(d) Thyroid hormones

T_3

T_4

(e) Metabolism of thyroid hormone

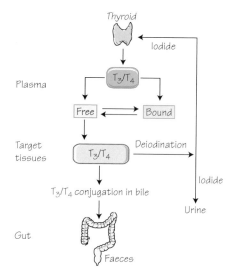

The Endocrine System at a Glance, 3rd edition. © Ben Greenstein and Diana Wood. Published 2011 by Blackwell Publishing Ltd.

Clinical scenario

Nodular thyroid disease is common, affecting approximately 5% of the female population over the age of 50. Women are affected more commonly than men and the incidence increases with age. A 59-year-old lady, Mrs RB, presented with a long history of a swelling in the anterior neck. This had gradually increased in size over the years and had now become quite obviously visible. She had no dysphagia or dyspnoea, the thyroid gland was not painful, she did not have a hoarse voice and there was no history of previous radiotherapy treatment to the neck. She had no symptoms to suggest abnormal thyroid hormone production and on examination she was clinically euthyroid. The thyroid gland was asymmetrically enlarged with a 3×4 cm nodule palpable in the right lobe together with three other palpable nodules. The gland moved freely on swallowing and there was no associated lymphadenopathy. Her thyroid function tests were normal as follows: fT_4 18.3 pmol/L; TSH 0.85 mU/L; thyroid antibodies negative. Thyroid ultrasound scanning revealed a multinodular goitre. Fine-needle aspiration of the dominant nodule was performed and cytology of the aspirate showed no evidence of malignant cells. She decided to undergo conservative management with regular clinical follow-up.

Clinical management of patients with nodular thyroid disease depends upon excluding the presence of malignant disease and then treating the goitre according to its size, patient preference and the likelihood of compression of other structures in the neck and mediastinum (Fig. 13a). In patients with compressive symptoms, CT scanning will reveal the extent of pressure on adjoining structures in the neck.

Thyroid gland: anatomy and structure

In humans, the thyroid gland is situated anteriorly in the neck (Fig. 13b), and its function is the synthesis and secretion of the thyroid hormones thyroxine (T_4) and tri-iodothyronine (T_3). These hormones are essential for normal development and growth and for homoeostasis in the body by regulating energy production. The parathyroid glands, which secrete parathyroid hormone (see Chapter 49) are embedded in the thyroid gland, and the parafollicular cells, which are scattered between the thyroid follicles, produce calcitonin (see Chapter 50). The human thyroid gland begins to develop at around 4 weeks after conception, and moves down the neck while forming its characteristic bilobular structure, which is completed by the third trimester.

In the normal adult, the gland has two lobes, weighs around 25 g and is situated close to the trachea (Fig. 13b). The gland is composed of well over a million clusters of cells, or follicles. These are spherical and consist of cells surrounding a central space containing a jelly-like substance known as colloid, whose function is to store thyroid hormones prior to their secretion. Each thyroid cell has three functions: (i) exocrine, because it secretes substances into the colloid; (ii) absorptive, because it takes up substances from the colloid by pinocytosis; and (iii) endocrine, because it secretes hormones directly into the bloodstream.

Thyroid hormones

Synthesis. The follicle cells have in their basement membrane an iodide-trapping mechanism which pumps dietary iodide into the cell (Fig.13c). The pump is very powerful, and the cell can concentrate iodide to 25–50 times its concentration in the plasma. Thyroid iodine content is normally around $600 \mu g/g$ tissue.

Uptake enhancers include: (i) TSH; (ii) iodine deficiency; (iii) TSH receptor antibodies; and (iv) autoregulation. **Uptake inhibitors** include: (i) I^- ions; (ii) cardiac glycosides (e.g. digoxin); (iii) thiocyanate (SCN^-); and (iv) perchlorate ($PClO_4^-$).

Inside the cell, iodide is rapidly oxidized by a peroxidase system to the more reactive iodine, which immediately reacts with tyrosine residues on a thyroid glycoprotein called thyroglobulin, to form mono-iodotyrosyl (T_1) or di-iodotyrosyl (T_2) thyroglobulin. These then couple to form tri-iodothyronine (T_3) or thyroxine (T_4) residues (Fig. 13d), still attached to thyroglobulin, which is stored in the colloid (i.e. $T_1 + T_2 = T_3$; $T_2 + T_2 = T_4$). This process is stimulated by TSH.

Under TSH stimulation, colloid droplets are taken back up into the cell cytoplasm by micropinocytosis, where they fuse with lysosomes and are proteolysed to release the residues from the glycoprotein. T_1 and T_2 are rapidly deiodinated by halogenases, and the liberated iodine is recycled in the follicle cell. Tri-iodothyronine and thyroxine (Fig. 13e) are released into the circulation, where they are bound to plasma proteins, including thyroxine-binding globulin (TGB), thyroxine-binding prealbumin (TBPA) and albumin (see Chapter 15). Most is bound and physiologically inactive, while only the free fraction is active.

Metabolism (Fig. 13e). The thyroid secretes a total of 80–100 μg of T_3 and T_4 per day, and the ratio of T_4:T_3 is about 20:1. Although both T_3 and T_4 circulate, the tissues obtain 90% of their T_3 by deiodinating T_4. Iodide liberated from thyroid hormone is excreted in the urine or is recirculated to the thyroid, where it is concentrated by the trapping mechanism. About one-third of T_4 leaving the plasma is conjugated with glucuronide or sulphate in the liver and excreted in the bile. A small proportion of the free T_4 is reabsorbed via the enterohepatic circulation. The half-life of T_4 in the plasma is about 6–7 days; that of T_3 is very much shorter, being about 1 day. T_3 is much more potent than is T_4.

Mechanism of action of thyroid hormone. There are multiple sites of action of T_3 in the cell. At the membrane, the hormone stimulates the Na^+/K^+–ATPase pump, resulting in increased uptake of amino acids and glucose, which causes calorigenesis (heat production). T_3 combines with specific receptors on mitochondria to generate energy and with intranuclear receptors which are transcription modulators, resulting in altered protein synthesis.

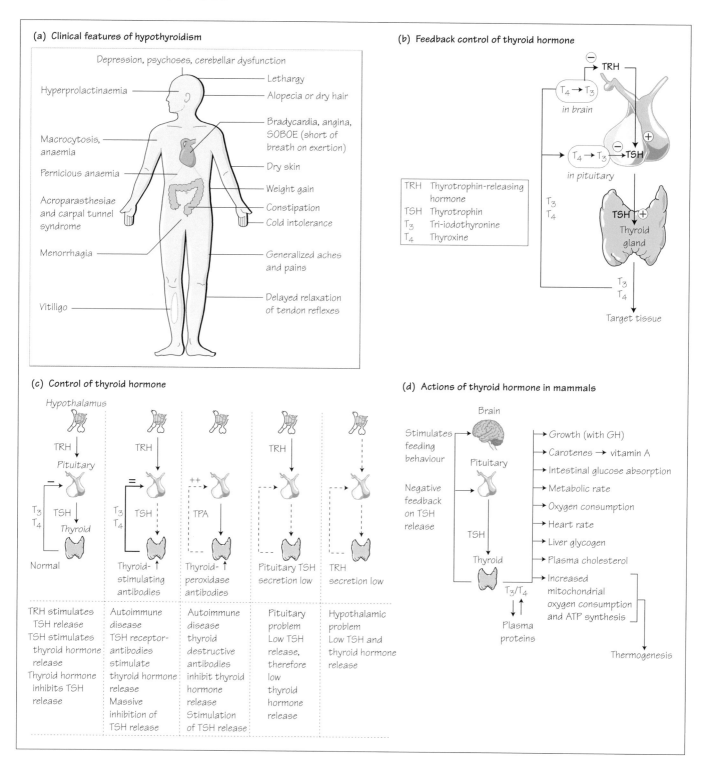

(a) Clinical features of hypothyroidism

Depression, psychoses, cerebellar dysfunction
Hyperprolactinaemia
Lethargy
Alopecia or dry hair
Bradycardia, angina, SOBOE (short of breath on exertion)
Macrocytosis, anaemia
Dry skin
Pernicious anaemia
Weight gain
Acroparasthesiae and carpal tunnel syndrome
Constipation
Cold intolerance
Menorrhagia
Generalized aches and pains
Delayed relaxation of tendon reflexes
Vitiligo

(b) Feedback control of thyroid hormone

TRH	Thyrotrophin-releasing hormone
TSH	Thyrotrophin
T_3	Tri-iodothyronine
T_4	Thyroxine

(c) Control of thyroid hormone

TRH stimulates TSH release	Autoimmune disease	Autoimmune disease	Pituitary problem	Hypothalamic problem
TSH stimulates thyroid hormone release	TSH receptor-antibodies stimulate thyroid hormone release	thyroid destructive antibodies inhibit thyroid hormone release	Low TSH release, therefore low thyroid hormone release	Low TSH and thyroid hormone release
Thyroid hormone inhibits TSH release	Massive inhibition of TSH release	Stimulation of TSH release		

(d) Actions of thyroid hormone in mammals

Stimulates feeding behaviour
Negative feedback on TSH release
Growth (with GH)
Carotenes → vitamin A
Intestinal glucose absorption
Metabolic rate
Oxygen consumption
Heart rate
Liver glycogen
Plasma cholesterol
Increased mitochondrial oxygen consumption and ATP synthesis
Plasma proteins
Thermogenesis

Clinical scenario

A 56-year-old woman, Miss TM, presented to her GP complaining of gaining weight, feeling cold and being tired all the time. Her hair and skin were very dry. On questioning she had noticed feeling out of breath more frequently, she was constipated and had generalized aches and pains with occasional tingling in her hands and feet. The GP thought she might be hypothyroid and on examination found her to have cool extremities with myxoedematous changes in the skin, her face was pale with periorbital puffiness, she was bradycardic and her tendon reflexes showed delayed relaxation. There was no goitre (Fig. 14a). The clinical diagnosis was confirmed biochemically when her thyroid function tests showed fT_4 of <2.0 pmol/L and TSH >75 mU/L. She had a high titre of thyroid peroxidase antibodies. She was started on thyroxine replacement therapy and her symptoms resolved over the next few weeks.

In the developed world, the vast majority of cases of primary hypothyroidism are caused by autoimmune disease or following treatment of thyrotoxicosis with radioactive iodine therapy or surgery. Autoimmune disease is either associated with destructive thyroid antibodies (antithyroid peroxidase antibodies) causing thyroid atrophy or, less commonly, with TSH-receptor-blocking antibodies causing the goitre of Hashimoto's disease. Drug-induced hypothyroidism may be seen, particularly in people taking lithium therapy and, rarely, congenital abnormalities of the thyroid or dyshormonogenesis may be found. Secondary hypothyroidism, characterized by low thyroxine and TSH concentrations and associated with disorders of the hypothalamo–pituitary axis, is rarely seen in general medical practice.

Control of thyroid hormone synthesis and secretion
Hypothalamic and pituitary control

Thyrotrophin-releasing hormone (**TRH**) is a tripeptide synthesized in the paraventricular and supraoptic nuclei in the hypothalamus and stored in the median eminence. The portal venous system transports TRH to the anterior pituitary where it stimulates *de novo* TSH synthesis and also releases TSH and prolactin. T_3 directly inhibits the TRH and TSH genes, thus regulating its own synthesis and release. TSH stimulates thyroid hormone synthesis and release at several points. In addition, a hypothalamic pulse regulator generates pulsatile release of TRH (Fig. 14b).

TSH belongs to a family of glycoproteins sharing common α and specific β subunits. The α-subunit is identical for LH, FSH, TSH and placental hCG. T_3 and T_4 inhibit synthesis and release of TSH. Conversely, falling levels of T_3 and T_4 stimulate TSH synthesis and release. TSH release is inhibited by other hormones and drugs, for example dopamine, the dopamine agonist bromocriptine, glucocorticoids and somatostatin. Hyperthyroidism will switch off TSH release altogether (Fig. 14c). Both TRH and TSH release may be impaired by hypothalamic or pituitary lesions or tumours.

Four mechanisms affect growth and function of the thyroid:

1 Circulating free thyroid hormones feed back at both hypothalamic and pituitary level to suppress TRH and TSH synthesis and release respectively (Fig. 14b).
2 Deiodinase enzymes in the pituitary modify the effects of T_3 and T_4. The hypothalamic and pituitary deiodinases remove iodine from T_4 to produce the active metabolite T_3. In hyperthyroidism, deiodinase activity is down-regulated to lessen the feedback effects of circulating T_4.
3 The thyroid cell autoregulates iodination. In hypothyroidism, T_3 is preferentially synthesized. In hyperthyroidism thyroid hormone synthesis is down-regulated.
4 TSH receptor antibodies may inhibit or stimulate thyroid function.

Actions of thyroid hormone (Fig. 14d)

Calorigenesis. Homoeotherms need to generate their own heat, and thyroid hormone does this by stimulating mitochondrial oxygen consumption and production of ATP, which is required for the sodium pump.

Carbohydrate and fat metabolism. Thyroid hormone has catabolic actions. It:

1 stimulates intestinal absorption of glucose;
2 stimulates hepatic glycogenolysis;
3 stimulates insulin breakdown;
4 potentiates the glycogenolytic actions of epinephrine.

Thyroid hormone is strongly lipolytic, both through a direct action and indirectly by potentiating the actions of other hormones, such as glucocorticoids, glucagon, growth hormone and epinephine. Thyroid hormone also increases oxidation of free fatty acids, which adds to the calorigenic effect. Thyroid hormone decreases plasma cholesterol by stimulating bile acid formation in the liver, which results in excretion in the faeces of cholesterol derivatives.

Growth and development. In humans, little T_3 or T_4 passes from the maternal to the fetal circulation. When the fetal thyroid is differentiated and functional, at 10–11 weeks' gestation, thyroid hormone becomes essential for normal differentiation and maturation of fetal tissues, although the hormone is not necessary for normal fetal growth. Therefore, babies with congenital hypothyroidism have retarded brain and skeletal maturation, but normal birth weight. In the brain, thyroid hormone causes myelinogenesis, protein synthesis and axonal ramification. It may act, in part, by stimulating production of nerve growth factor. Thyroid hormone is essential for normal growth hormone (GH) production. In addition, GH is ineffective in the absence of thyroid hormone.

Mechanism of action of thyroid hormone

At the cell membrane, T_3 stimulates the Na^+/K^+–ATPase pump, resulting in increased uptake of amino acids and glucose, which causes calorigenesis. T_3 combines with specific receptors on mitochondria to generate energy and with intranuclear receptors which are transcription modulators, resulting in altered protein synthesis. There is evidence for different isoforms of the receptor, whose expression profiles vary with age and tissue (Chapter 4).

(a) Clinical features of thyrotoxicosis

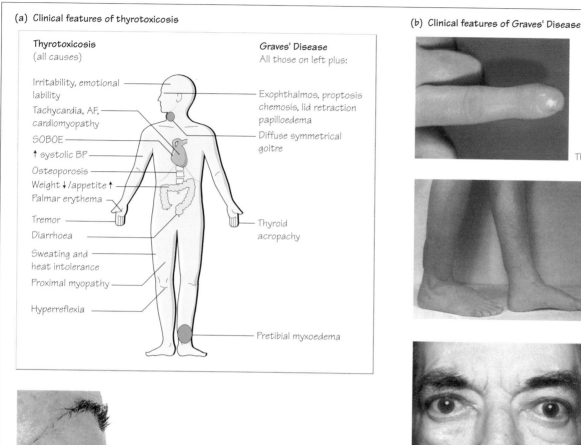

Thyrotoxicosis
(all causes)

Irritability, emotional lability

Tachycardia, AF, cardiomyopathy

SOBOE

↑ systolic BP

Osteoporosis

Weight ↓/appetite ↑

Palmar erythema

Tremor

Diarrhoea

Sweating and heat intolerance

Proximal myopathy

Hyperreflexia

Graves' Disease
All those on left plus:

Exophthalmos, proptosis chemosis, lid retraction papilloedema

Diffuse symmetrical goitre

Thyroid acropachy

Pretibial myxoedema

(b) Clinical features of Graves' Disease

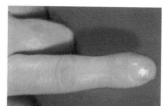

Thyroid acropachy

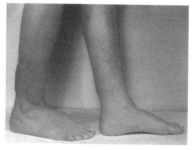

Pre-tibial myxoedema

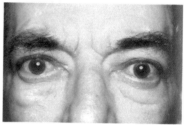

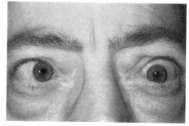

Left VIth nerve palsy

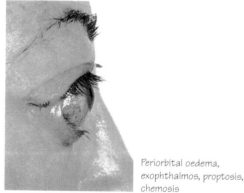

Periorbital oedema, exophthalmos, proptosis, chemosis

Clinical scenario

Mrs JA, a 41-year-old part-time nurse presented to her GP with a 6-month history of weight loss of 10 kg. On questioning she was eating well but complained of diarrhoea. She had also noticed that she felt exhausted and had developed insomnia. On further questioning she admitted to feeling increasingly hot and shaky and to having muscle weakness of the legs, particularly climbing stairs. She was normally well and had not seen the doctor since her last pregnancy 8 years before. A blood test showed the following results: free T_4 49.7 pmol/L; total T_4 225 nmol/L; TSH <0.01 mU/L.

She was referred to an endocrinologist at the local hospital where initial investigations confirmed a diagnosis of Graves' disease. She was treated with carbimazole and propranolol for the first month of treatment followed by carbimazole alone. Subsequently, after discussing the therapeutic options, she opted to have ^{131}I therapy which was given as an outpatient when she had become euthyroid. She was followed up at regular outpatient visits and 6 months later complained of lethargy, weight gain and feeling cold all the time. Clinically she had features of hypothyroidism and blood tests were as follows: free T_4 4.5 pmol/L; TSH 25.7 mU/L. The endocrinologist commenced thyroid hormone replacement therapy and 3 months later she was well and her blood tests were normal.

Introduction

There are a number of causes of hyperthyroidism but over 90% of cases are accounted for by autoimmune thyrotoxicosis (Graves' disease, approximately 75%), toxic multinodular goitre (approximately 15%) and solitary toxic adenoma (approximately 5%). Transient thyrotoxicosis may be associated with thyroiditis and certain drugs may be responsible, particularly amiodarone. Very rarely patients present with thyrotoxicosis secondary to TSH-secreting tumours of the pituitary, pituitary thyroid hormone resistance syndrome, extrathyroidal hormone excess or secondary to thyroid carcinoma.

Clinically, the features of thyrotoxicosis may be divided into those caused by thyroid hormone excess and seen in all cases of hyperthyroidism and those associated with autoimmunity and seen in patients with Graves' disease only (Fig. 15a and b; Table 15.1). Treatment is either with antithyroid drugs (alone or in combination with thyroxine replacement therapy), radioactive iodine ablation using ^{131}I or surgery. Choice of treatment depends on the underlying cause and may be influenced by the patient's age, other coexisting disease, particularly in the elderly, or the presence of thyroid-associated ophthalmopathy.

Thyroid function tests
Thyroid hormone measurement

Only about 1% of thyroid hormones are in the metabolically active 'free' state as both T_4 and T_3 are tightly bound to transport proteins in the plasma (Chapter 13). Assays of 'total' T_4 or T_3 measure mainly the protein-bound hormone. This may be affected in a number of ways by conditions affecting protein concentration. Thus spuriously high total T_4 measurements will occur in pregnancy and in women taking the oral contraceptive pill as estrogen increases thyroxine binding globulin (TBG) synthesis. Inappropriately low measurements may be found in individuals with congenital TBG deficiency or severe liver disease.

Assays of 'free' thyroid hormones are now widely available and are not generally affected by changes in plasma binding protein concentrations.

Thyroid stimulating hormone measurement

Measurement of TSH is the most widely used thyroid function test. It is less subject to assay interference and reliably predicts thyroid function in accordance with the principles of negative feedback. Thus in hyperthyroidism the TSH concentration is undetectable. In primary hypothyroidism, TSH concentrations are elevated and in secondary hypothyroidism the low free T_4 level is accompanied by low TSH concentrations.

Other biochemical tests of thyroid function, such as TRH tests, have been used only rarely since the advent of highly sensitive TSH assays.

Thyroid imaging

Biochemical tests of thyroid function may be supplemented by imaging techniques to investigate thyroid structure and function:
• **Thyroid ultrasonography** will reveal the presence of single or multiple nodules and cysts. Needle aspiration for cytology or cyst drainage and thyroid biopsy may be conducted under ultrasound control.
• **Thyroid scintigraphy** or radionuclide imaging is helpful in the diagnosis of thyroiditis, when isotope uptake is greatly diminished in contrast to the uniform increase seen in thyrotoxicosis. A clinically solitary nodule may be revealed as a 'cold' nodule on scanning, requiring further investigation for possible malignant disease.

Thyroid cancer

Thyroid cancer usually presents as a swelling in the thyroid gland. It is a relatively rare malignancy and the majority of thyroid nodules will prove to be benign. Investigations include fine-needle aspiration cytology, with or without thyroid scintigraphy. Most malignancies are papillary carcinomas; other tumours include the more aggressive follicular carcinomas and rapidly progressive anaplastic lesions. Medullary thyroid carcinomas arising in thyroid C cells may be found in isolation or as part of the MEN 2 syndrome (see Chapter 50).

Table 15.1 Clinical features of thyrotoxicosis

Features of hyperthyroidism		Features of Graves' disease
Common	*Less common*	*Features of hyperthyroidism plus*
Weight loss despite normal/increased appetite	Weight gain	Diffuse symmetrical goitre with bruit
Diarrhoea	Anorexia	Exophthalmos, proptosis
Breathlessness on exertion	Thirst	Chemosis
Palpitations, sinus tachycardia	Vomiting	Eyelid retraction
Irritability and emotional lability	Raised systolic BP with increased pulse pressure	Excess watering of eyes
Tremor	Atrial fibrillation	Corneal ulceration
Muscle weakness	Cardiomyopathy, cardiac failure	Diplopia and ophthalmoplegia
Fatigue	Proximal myopathy, bulbar myopathy	Papilloedema, loss of visual acuity
Hyper-reflexia	Palmar erythema	Thyroid acropachy (clubbing of the digits)
Lid lag	Onycholysis	Localized (especially pretibial) myxoedema
Oedema	Subfertility, spontaneous abortion	
Sweating, heat intolerance	Gynaecomastia	
Pruritis	Osteoporosis	

Adrenal gland: I Adrenal medulla

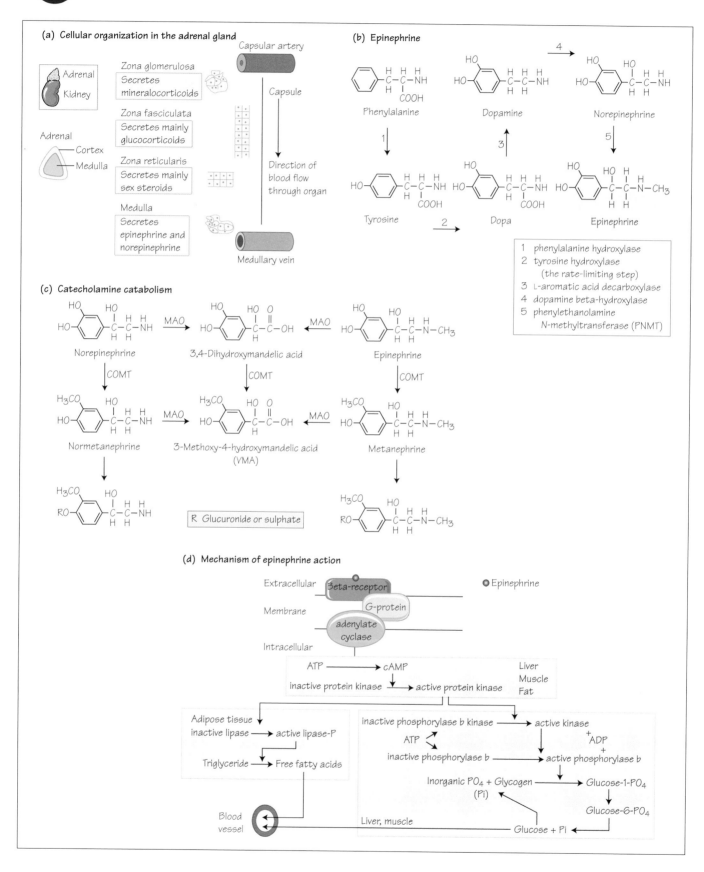

Clinical scenario

A 32-year-old accountant, Mr PT, went to the Occupational Health Department at his workplace as he had been experiencing headaches and palpitations for the last few months. These had become increasingly frequent and his colleagues had noticed that he became extremely pale at the times he complained of palpitations. At the time of these episodes he had a bizarre sensation of extreme anxiety and fear of death. There was nothing to find on examination apart from an elevated blood pressure of 180/105. There was no significant family history.

The occupational health physician was sufficiently concerned to refer him to the local Endocrine Department. Investigations there revealed elevated levels of plasma and urine metanephrines. Abdominal MRI scans and radioisotope scanning using iodine-labelled meta-iodobenzyl guanidine (MIBG) demonstrated a 5 × 6 cm mass in the region of the right adrenal gland consistent with a phaeochromocytoma. He was treated with the α-adrenoceptor-blocking drug phenoxybenzamine with the later addition of the β-blocker propranolol prior to surgery 6 weeks later. At operation the phaeochromocytoma was removed and he made an uneventful recovery.

Phaeochromocytomas are rare tumours of the adrenal medulla secreting catecholamines, usually norepinephrine The majority are sporadic, benign lesions although approximately 10% are familial and 10% malignant. In approximately 10% of cases they are extramedullary, making localization difficult. Phaeochromocytomas may be part of the Multiple Endocrine Neoplasia Type 2 syndrome (MEN 2; Chapter 50).

The adrenal glands

The adrenal glands lie just above the kidneys (Fig. 16a), and can be divided on anatomical and functional grounds into two main suborgans: (1) the adrenal cortex, which secretes the steroid hormones; and (2) the adrenal medulla, a modified ganglion, which secretes the catecholamines epinephrine (EP) and norepinephrine (NE).

Adrenal medulla

Catecholamine synthesis (Fig. 16b). The adrenal medullary chromaffin cells can be distinguished as EP-storing and NE-storing cells.

EP and NE are stored in granules, together with a protein, chromogranin, and adenosine triphosphate (ATP). When exocytosed, the granule releases all its contents.

Metabolism (Fig. 16c). Catecholamines are metabolized extracellularly and in the liver by catecholamine-*O*-methyltransferase (COMT), and intracellularly by monoamine oxidase (MAO). MAO is localized close to the adrenoceptors where EP and NE act. Catecholamine action is not terminated by enzymes, however, but through reuptake into the cell from which they were released. VMA is excreted in the urine. In sympathetic nerves, NE feeds back onto presynaptic α-2 receptors, which limit further release of NE. Metabolites are measured in urine and are diagnostic in phaeochromocytoma.

Actions of epinephrine

Epinephrine has been called the hormone of 'flight or fight'. Stressors cause an immediate release of EP, which prepares the body for extraordinary physical and mental exertion (Table 16.1). Surface vasculature shuts down by the constriction of arteriolar tissue through the mediation of α-1 receptors, thus limiting potential blood loss through injury; in contrast, the vasculature to the muscular beds opens up through the activation of the β-2 receptors. Dilation of bronchioles increases the efficiency of oxygen intake in unit time, and glucose mobilization is enhanced through the stimulation of **glucagon** release and the inhibition of **insulin** release. Dilation of the radial muscles of the iris in the eye increases the availability of light to the retina, and the contraction of the splenic capsule releases blood cells into the circulation. Through β-1 receptors in the heart, contractility is greatly increased. Epinephrine promotes lipolysis and thermogenesis through β-3 receptors. EP also increases mental alertness, although the exact mechanism is unknown.

Mechanism of epinephrine action (Fig. 16d). An example of EP action is the mobilization of energy in the form of glucose. EP also acts on β receptors in muscle to inhibit release of amino acids, thus reducing the rate of muscle proteolysis. This mechanism may be important in the fight or flight response, when muscle would be spared from providing energy. Although little NE is released from the adrenal medulla, it is the major neurotransmitter of the sympathetic nervous system which is activated during fight or flight.

Table 16.1 Actions of epinephrine

Site of action	Effect	Receptor
Heart	Increased rate and force of contraction	β-1
Blood vessels		
Skin		
Mucous membranes	Contract	α-1
Splanchnic bed		
Skeletal muscle	Dilate	β-2
Respiratory system	Bronchodilation	β-2
Gastrointestinal tract		
Smooth muscle	Relax	α-2
Sphincters	Contract	α-1
Blood		
Coagulation time	Decreased	
Red blood count (Haemoglobin)	Increased	
Plasma protein		
Metabolism		
Insulin release	Decreased	α-2
Glucagon release		β-2
Thermogenesis	Increased	β-3
Lipolysis		β-3
Eye-radial muscle	Contract	α-1
Smooth muscle		
Splenic capsule		
Uterus	Contract	α-1
Vas deferens		

17 Adrenal gland: II Adrenocortical hormones

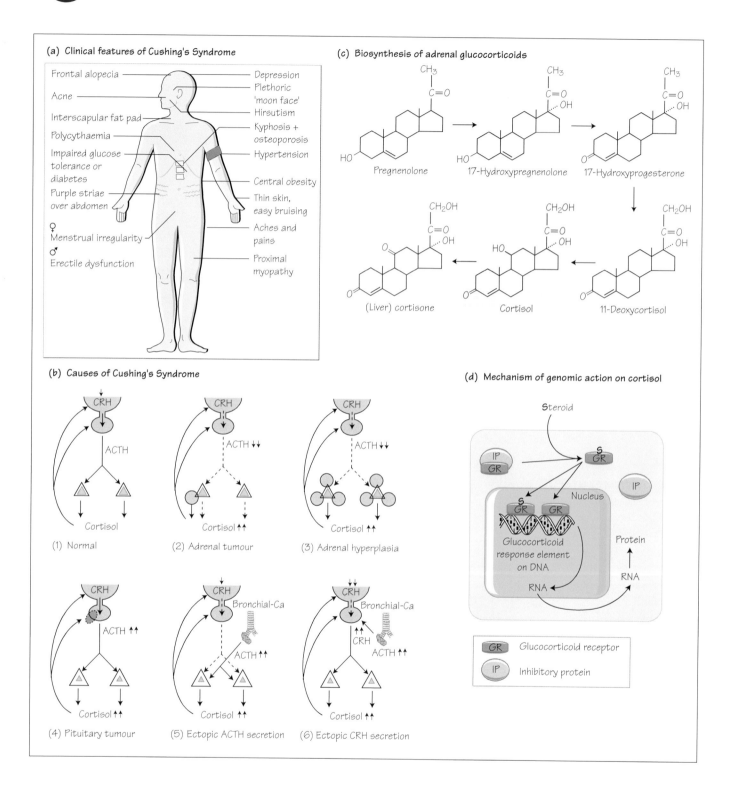

(a) Clinical features of Cushing's Syndrome

Frontal alopecia
Acne
Interscapular fat pad
Polycythaemia
Impaired glucose tolerance or diabetes
Purple striae over abdomen
♀ Menstrual irregularity
♂ Erectile dysfunction

Depression
Plethoric 'moon face'
Hirsutism
Kyphosis + osteoporosis
Hypertension
Central obesity
Thin skin, easy bruising
Aches and pains
Proximal myopathy

(c) Biosynthesis of adrenal glucocorticoids

Pregnenolone → 17-Hydroxypregnenolone → 17-Hydroxyprogesterone

(Liver) cortisone ← Cortisol ← 11-Deoxycortisol

(b) Causes of Cushing's Syndrome

(1) Normal — ACTH — Cortisol
(2) Adrenal tumour — ACTH ↓↓ — Cortisol ↑↑
(3) Adrenal hyperplasia — ACTH ↓↓ — Cortisol ↑↑
(4) Pituitary tumour — ACTH ↑↑ — Cortisol ↑↑
(5) Ectopic ACTH secretion — Bronchial-Ca — ACTH ↑↑ — Cortisol ↑↑
(6) Ectopic CRH secretion — Bronchial-Ca — CRH — ACTH ↑↑ — Cortisol ↑↑

(d) Mechanism of genomic action on cortisol

Steroid
Nucleus
Glucocorticoid response element on DNA
Protein
RNA

GR Glucocorticoid receptor
IP Inhibitory protein

Table 17.1 Clinical features of Cushing's syndrome of whatever cause in order of frequency

Plethoric, 'moon face'
Central obesity
Impaired glucose tolerance or diabetes
Hypertension
Menstrual irregularity (women), erectile dysfunction (men)
Osteoporosis
Purple striae, particularly over abdomen, and tendency to bruise easily
Proximal myopathy
Hirsutism and frontal alopecia (women, indicating androgen excess)
Ankle oedema
Interscapular fat pad
Acne
Musculoskeletal aches and pains
Depression
Poor wound healing
Kyphosis secondary to osteoporosis
Polycythaemia

Clinical background

Cushing's syndrome is the name given to the clinical symptoms and physical signs induced by glucocorticoid excess (Fig. 17a; Table 17.1). It may be caused by excess adrenocorticotrophic hormone (ACTH) secretion by a pituitary tumour resulting in bilateral adrenocortical hyperplasia or by adrenal cortical tumours such as benign adenomas or malignant carcinomas (Fig. 17b). Patients with ACTH-dependent Cushing's syndrome and adrenal carcinomas often demonstrate coexisting androgen hypersecretion, accounting for some of the clinical features of the syndrome. Adrenal Cushing's syndrome can be diagnosed by finding elevated plasma cortisol concentrations with loss of the normal diurnal variation and failure to suppress following short and (usually) long dexamethasone suppression tests in the presence of undetectable plasma ACTH concentrations. Adrenal tumours are visualized by MRI or CT scanning and their treatment is surgical, followed by adrenolytic chemotherapy in those patients with malignant disease.

Adrenocortical hormones

The adrenal cortex synthesizes and secretes steroid hormones. The predominant hormones are:
• **Cortisol**: glucocorticoid action on carbohydrate metabolism and the response to stress. Excess glucocorticoids have catabolic effects on protein metabolism.
• **Aldosterone**: regulates salt and water homeostasis.
• **Androgens**: testosterone, androstenedione, 17 hydroxyprogesterone and dehydroepiandrosterone sulphate (DHEAS) all have effects on the maintenance of secondary sexual characteristics. Excess androgen production results in virilization in the female.

Biosynthesis of glucocorticoids

Pregnenolone is formed from cholesterol (CH) by side-chain cleavage catalysed by the desmolase enzyme system. CH is mainly transported in the blood in low density lipoprotein (LDL). The LDL consists of an inner hydrophobic core of CH esters and triglyceride, surrounded by a monolayer of polar phospholipid and apoproteins. One of the apoproteins, apolipoprotein-E (APO-E), binds to receptors (LP receptors) on the plasma membrane of the adrenal cell, resulting in an ACTH-stimulated transport of CH into the cell. This sequence of actions is termed the LDL receptor pathway.

LDL has been linked with atherosclerotic disease, and the genetic disorder known as type III lipoproteinaemia, associated with premature atherosclerotic disease, possibly occurs because of the nature of the APO-E in these individuals. Their APO-E does not bind with normal affinity to the LP receptor.

After pregnenolone is released from the mitochondria, it is further metabolized in the smooth endoplasmic reticulum, where the double bond is switched from position 5 in the B ring to position 4 in the A ring, and the hydroxyl (OH) group at position 3 is oxidized to a keto group. Cortisol is formed through hydroxylation at the 11 position (Fig. 17c). Cortisol is the major glucocorticoid in humans, although further metabolism to another glucocorticoid, cortisone, occurs in the liver.

Synthesis of adrenal androgens

Adrenal androgens are biosynthesized from androstenedione, which is formed from 17-hydroxyprogesterone by the cleavage of the C17 side chain, and hydroxylation at C17. Androstenedione, an adrenal androgen, can be formed through isomerization at the C4–C5 positions, as described previously for glucocorticoids, or after cleavage at C17.

Synthesis of adrenal estrogens

Estrogens are formed from testosterone and androstenedione by aromatization of the A ring. The term 'aromatization' refers to the formation of alternating double bonds in the six-membered ring. The conversion is achieved through the removal of the methyl group at C19, and further oxidation.

Neither the adrenal androgens nor the estrogens are normally produced in sufficient quantities to support reproductive function; the testis and ovary, respectively, are required for that purpose, but adrenal androgens and estrogens, and particularly the former, do become pathologically significant if produced in too high a concentration.

Mechanism of action of cortisol

Cortisol, like many other steroid hormones, passes freely into the cytoplasm where it combines with a receptor (Fig. 17d). The glucocorticoid–receptor complex is translocated to the nucleus where it binds to specific response elements, resulting in RNA and protein synthesis, although transcription may sometimes be inhibited. There is evidence that some of the rapid actions of cortisol, for example on feedback in the brain and pituitary gland, are through cell membrane receptors for cortisol.

18 Adrenal gland: III Adrenocorticotrophic hormone (ACTH)

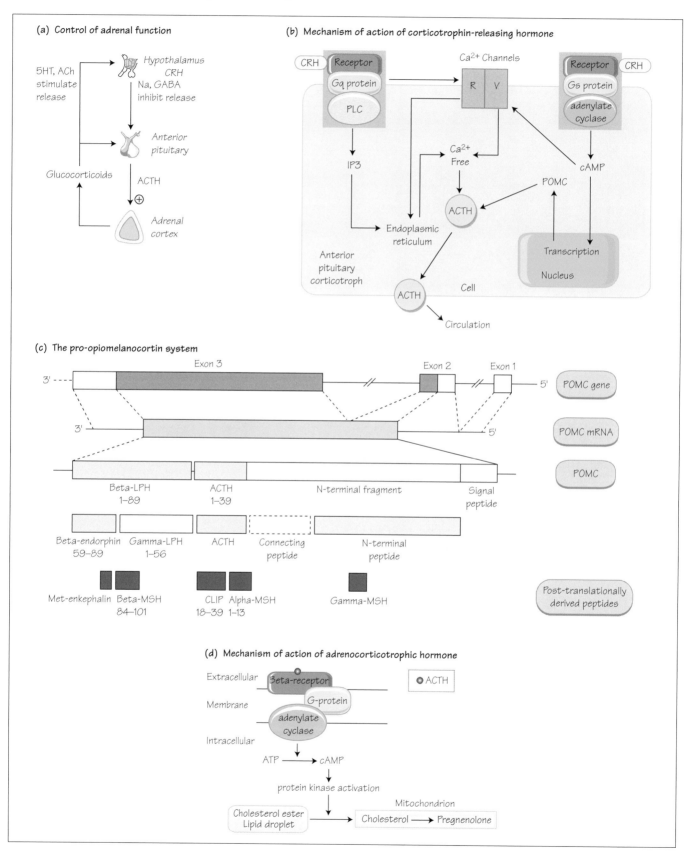

(a) Control of adrenal function

(b) Mechanism of action of corticotrophin-releasing hormone

(c) The pro-opiomelanocortin system

(d) Mechanism of action of adrenocorticotrophic hormone

Clinical scenario

A 28-year-old interior designer, ZL, presented to her GP with a 12-month history of change in her appearance, excess facial hair growth and irregular, scanty periods. She had noticed that her cheeks were becoming fatter and that she was always red in the face, with the onset of greasy skin and acne more latterly. She had marked hair growth over her chin and upper lip. On questioning, she had gained weight 'round the middle' and noticed the development of red stretch marks on her abdomen. She generally felt very low about things. Physical examination suggested that she had Cushing's syndrome and she was referred to the local endocrine clinic. When she arrived there, the above features were noted plus a marked proximal myopathy. Investigations revealed elevated urinary free cortisol levels, plasma cortisol concentrations of 1059 nmol/L at 0900h and 1003 nmol/L at midnight. The ACTH concentration at 0900h was 230 ng/L. Pituitary MRI scanning suggested an abnormality in the left side of the gland, and this was supported by bilateral catheterization of the petrosal sinuses with multiple ACTH measurements. She underwent trans-sphenoidal surgery with removal of a pituitary adenoma which stained strongly for ACTH on immunohistochemical testing. Postoperatively her symptoms resolved associated with normalization of her pituitary function.

Adrenocorticotrophic hormone

Control of adrenocorticotrophic hormone (ACTH) secretion. ACTH is synthesized in the anterior pituitary corticotroph cells and is released on stimulation of the corticotroph cell by the hypothalamic peptide corticotrophin-releasing hormone (CRH; Fig. 18a). Human CRH is a peptide containing 41 amino acids and is sometimes referred to as CRH-41. It is a potent releaser of ACTH, both *in vivo* and *in vitro*. CRH-41 is widely distributed throughout the brain but the greatest concentration is in the hypothalamus, within the parvocellular neurones of the paraventricular nucleus (see Chapter 5). These neurones project many fibres to the median eminence, where they release CRH into the portal circulation. Other peptides, notably vasopressin, may physiologically potentiate the ACTH-releasing action of CRH. The interaction between CRH and vasopressin (here abbreviated to AVP, because it is structurally arginine–vasopressin) involves their interaction with receptors on the membrane of the anterior corticotroph cell (Fig. 18b).

AVP activates the IP3 second messenger system, which opens receptor-gated calcium channels. CRH acts through the adenylate cyclase–cAMP second messenger system, and opens voltage-gated calcium channels. The increased free intracellular Ca^{2+} stimulates ACTH release. ACTH synthesis is stimulated through CRH-mediated increased expression of the pro-opiomelanocortin (POMC) gene, which contains the genetic information required for synthesis of ACTH, and the hormone melanocyte-stimulating hormone.

CRH release from the hypothalamus is stimulated by the neurotransmitters acetylcholine and serotonin (5HT). It is inhibited by gamma-aminobutyric acid (GABA) and norepinephrine (NE). CRH and ACTH release are inhibited by the glucocorticoids in a negative-feedback loop; this loop is useful in testing the integrity of the hypothalamic–hypophyseal–adrenal axis (Chapter 17).

The pro-opiomelanocortin (POMC) system. Anterior pituitary corticotrophs synthesize a glycoprotein which contains the complete amino acid sequences of ACTH, β-lipotrophin (β-LPH), melanocyte-stimulating hormone (MSH), met-enkephalin and a number of other peptides (Fig. 18c). POMC has a 26 amino acid signal sequence, followed by three main structural domains, namely: (i) ACTH; (ii) β-LPH at the C-terminal; and (iii) the N-terminal sequence pro- γ-MSH (for which no biological role has yet been found). POMC is first cleaved to give β-LPH and ACTH, which is still attached to the N-terminal fragment. In anterior pituitary corticotrophs, ACTH is released at the second cleavage. A number of molecules of β-LPH are cleaved to give β-endorphin and γ-LPH. It appears that on stimulation of the corticotroph with CRH, all the POMC-derived peptides are secreted together, suggesting that they are held together in the same secretory granule, and supporting the idea that they all derive from POMC. In species which possess a functional pituitary intermediate lobe (e.g. the rat, but not the adult human), further cleavage of many of the peptides occurs; for example the cleavage of ACTH into $ACTH_{1-13}$, which is α-N acetylated to yield α-MSH and $ACTH_{18-39}$.

Mechanism of adrenocorticotrophic hormone action. ACTH binds to high affinity membrane receptors on the adrenal cell, activating the adenylate cyclase system (Fig.18d). Maximum stimulation of steroidogenesis can be achieved with a plasma concentration of around 3 ng/L of ACTH. Increased intracellular concentrations of cAMP enhance the transport of cholesterol to a mitochondrial side chain cleavage enzyme, and they activate cholesterol ester hydroxylase. In addition, RNA and protein synthesis in the cell are stimulated, and there is a net increase in adrenal protein phosphorylation.

ACTH and calcium channels. ACTH promotes cortisol secretion partly through stimulation of Ca^{2+} channel production on cortisol-releasing cells, and this finding may have important implications for future modification of cortisol release.

ACTH, CRH and the immune system. CRH stimulates B cell proliferation and NK activity. It also stimulates IL-1, IL-2 and IL-6 production. CRH receptors have been found on immune cells. Injection of CRH directly into the cerebral ventricles inhibits immune function. CRH injected intracerebroventricularly has largely inhibitory effects on immune function. ACTH has been shown to inhibit antibody production to some extent and it modulates B cell function.

19 Adrenal gland: IV Cortisol and androgens

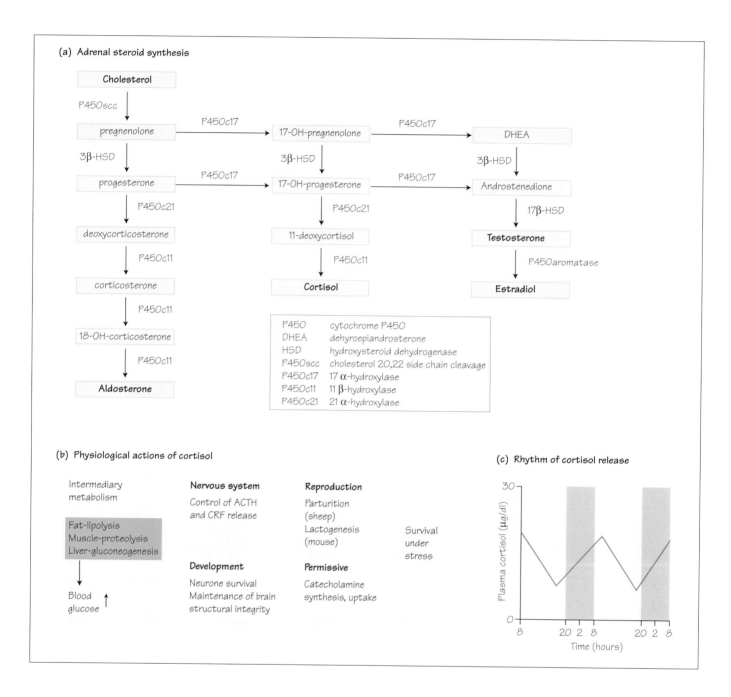

(a) Adrenal steroid synthesis

Cholesterol → (P450scc) → pregnenolone → (P450c17) → 17-OH-pregnenolone → (P450c17) → DHEA

pregnenolone → (3β-HSD) → progesterone

17-OH-pregnenolone → (3β-HSD) → 17-OH-progesterone

DHEA → (3β-HSD) → Androstenedione

progesterone → (P450c17) → 17-OH-progesterone → (P450c17) → Androstenedione

progesterone → (P450c21) → deoxycorticosterone → (P450c11) → corticosterone → (P450c11) → 18-OH-corticosterone → (P450c11) → Aldosterone

17-OH-progesterone → (P450c21) → 11-deoxycortisol → (P450c11) → Cortisol

Androstenedione → (17β-HSD) → Testosterone → (P450aromatase) → Estradiol

P450   cytochrome P450
DHEA   dehyroepiandrosterone
HSD   hydroxysteroid dehydrogenase
P450scc   cholesterol 20,22 side chain cleavage
P450c17   17 α-hydroxylase
P450c11   11 β-hydroxylase
P450c21   21 α-hydroxylase

(b) Physiological actions of cortisol

Intermediary metabolism

Fat-lipolysis
Muscle-proteolysis
Liver-gluconeogenesis

↓

Blood glucose ↑

Nervous system

Control of ACTH and CRF release

Development

Neurone survival
Maintenance of brain structural integrity

Reproduction

Parturition (sheep)
Lactogenesis (mouse)

Permissive

Catecholamine synthesis, uptake

Survival under stress

(c) Rhythm of cortisol release

Plasma cortisol (μg/dl) vs Time (hours)

Clinical background

Congenital adrenal hyperplasia (CAH) describes a number of conditions arising from absence or impaired function of enzymes in the adrenal steroidogenic pathway. Over 95% of cases represent deficiencies in the 21-hydroxylase enzyme (21-OHD, 'classical' CAH), with abnormalities of 11β-hydroxylase, 3β-hydroxysteroid dehydrogenase, 17α-hydroxylase and 20,22-desmolase deficiencies also being described (Fig. 19a).

The clinical features of CAH depend upon the genetic basis of the disorder in individuals. Thus, complete deletion of the 21-OH gene will produce the full-blown effects of CAH, whereas gene mutations may be responsible for lesser clinical features corresponding to impaired enzyme action. The clinical features of CAH can be surmised by consideration of the steroidogenic pathway. In classical 21-OHD with severe enzyme deficiency, androgen production is increased alongside decreased synthesis of cortisol and aldosterone, leading to the typical clinical features of a newborn with ambiguous genitalia. In females this is generally identified at birth, so that early treatment prevents the onset of salt-losing crisis secondary to mineralocorticoid deficiency. In male babies, this may present as failure to thrive, and subsequent vomiting, diarrhoea and circulatory collapse are the presenting clinical features. Milder variants of classical 21-OHD may present in childhood with virilization and precocious puberty. Those with 'non-classical' forms of the disease may not present until early adulthood, usually young women with irregular menses and hirsutism. Treatment of CAH is by glucocorticoid replacement therapy, thereby restoring the negative feedback in the pituitary–adrenal axis and lowering the ACTH drive to androgen production. In young women with non-classical CAH this may be combined with antiandrogen therapy.

The molecular genetics of CAH have been the subject of much investigation. Prenatal diagnosis can be offered to affected families, either by chorionic villous sampling in the early stages of pregnancy or later amniocentesis. Prenatal treatment with glucocorticoids can prevent the virilization of a female fetus.

Physiological actions of cortisol

Physiologically, cortisol affects intermediary metabolism, the nervous system and some processes related to reproduction. It permits other chemical mediators to act and, overall, it enables the organism to survive under stress (Fig. 19b; Table 19.1).

Intermediary metabolism. Cortisol increases the synthesis of a number of enzymes which play key roles in hepatic gluconeogenesis. This is an anabolic action of cortisol. In adipose tissue (fat) and skeletal muscle, however, cortisol is catabolic, that is it causes a breakdown of body tissues in order to mobilize energy. In these tissues, glucose uptake is inhibited and another substrate for adenosine triphosphate (ATP) production is found through proteolysis in muscle and lipolysis in fat. The free fatty acids released from muscle and fat travel to the liver, where they are taken up and utilized as substrates for gluconeogenesis. The net result is increased glucose or hyperglycaemia.

Nervous system. Adrenocorticotrophic hormone (ACTH) and cortisol are synthesized and released in a diurnal rhythm (Fig. 19c). The rhythm is determined by the interaction with the external environment, particularly the light–dark cycle and sleep patterns, and this implicates the brain. The brain releases corticotrophin releasing hormone (CRH), which in turn releases ACTH, which stimulates glucocorticoid release. Glucocorticoids feed back to the anterior pituitary and hypothalamus to limit ACTH and CRH release, respectively, through their intracellular receptors and possibly through membrane glucocorticoid receptors. The application of the synthetic glucocorticoid dexamethasone abolishes the CRH stimulation of ACTH. The diurnal rhythm of glucocorticoid secretion reflects a similar rhythm of ACTH secretion. The rhythms are regulated by a 'biological clock', which may reside in the suprachiasmatic area of the brain (Chapter 5). The mechanism that causes the

Table 19.1 Actions of glucocorticoids

Tissue	Action
Liver	Gluconeogenesis to increase glycogen stores
Fat	Lipolysis
Parturition	Fetal cortisol initiates parturition in sheep
Skeletal muscle	Atrophy through loss of protein
Connective tissue	Inhibition of growth
Immune system and lymphoid tissue	Suppression of immune system, atrophy of lymphoid tissue, mitosis inhibited, anti-inflammatory
ACTH	Inhibition of release from anterior pituitary gland
Water metabolism	Water retention by inhibiting glomerular filtration

rhythm is thus inbuilt, but may be synchronized by exogenous (outside) influences such as light. This is particularly important in the case of seasonal breeding animals, where day length may determine the onset and offset of reproductive activity.

Glucocorticoids influence neuronal development in the fetal and neonatal brain. Administration of glucocorticoids to neonatal rats results in a reduction in both the basal level and the diurnal rhythm of ACTH and glucocorticoid release in the adult. This suggests that endogenous glucocorticoids may play a part in the normal development of the CRH–ACTH axis. In the adult rat, adrenalectomy (removal of the adrenal gland) results in the loss of neurones in specific regions of the hippocampus, an area of the brain concerned with memory, learning and the functioning of the hypothalamic–pituitary systems. Concurrent administration of glucocorticoids with adrenalectomy prevents neuronal loss, suggesting that glucocorticoids help to maintain cellular and structural integrity in specific areas of the brain.

Permissive actions and stress. Glucocorticoids allow other hormones to exert certain effects. For example: they are required for catecholamine synthesis and reuptake into nerve; they enable the process of catecholamine-stimulated fat mobilization; and, through their effects on gluconeogenesis, they permit the body to maintain its temperature and its response to stress. The body's response to stress has been termed the General Adaptation Syndrome (GAS). Three main phases have been postulated: (i) alarm reaction; followed by (ii) resistance; and then by (iii) exhaustion. The alarm reaction is the initial release of epinephrine from the adrenal medulla and the release of norepinephrine from sympathetic nerve terminals. At the same time, glucocorticoids are released, and these permit the catecholamines to act. Their onset of action is slower than that of the catecholamines, so they provide a continued resistance to stress. If stress is prolonged, this leads to exhaustion, characterized by muscle wasting, atrophy of tissues of the immune system, gastric ulceration, hyperglycaemia and vascular damage.

20 Adrenal gland: V Aldosterone

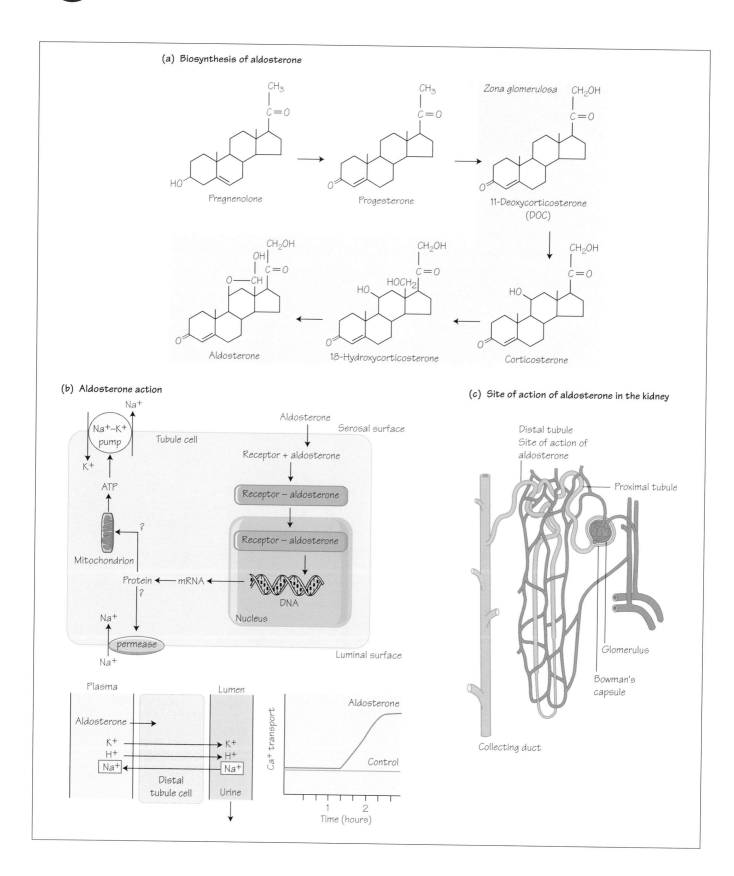

(a) Biosynthesis of aldosterone

Pregnenolone

Progesterone

Zona glomerulosa

11-Deoxycorticosterone (DOC)

Corticosterone

18-Hydroxycorticosterone

Aldosterone

(b) Aldosterone action

Na^+

Na^+–K^+ pump

K^+

ATP

Mitochondrion

Tubule cell

Aldosterone

Serosal surface

Receptor + aldosterone

Receptor – aldosterone

Receptor – aldosterone

DNA

Nucleus

Protein ← mRNA

Na^+

permease

Na^+

Luminal surface

Plasma

Lumen

Aldosterone

K^+ → K^+

H^+ → H^+

Na^+ ← Na^+

Distal tubule cell

Urine

Ca^+ transport

Aldosterone

Control

Time (hours)

(c) Site of action of aldosterone in the kidney

Distal tubule
Site of action of aldosterone

Proximal tubule

Glomerulus

Bowman's capsule

Collecting duct

Clinical scenario

42-year-old Mr J-P T was referred to the hypertension clinic of his local hospital as his GP had established that he had hypertension in the order of 180–190/105–110. An ECG showed evidence of early left ventricular hypertrophy but fundoscopy was normal. Blood tests were taken and the results showed Na^+ 144 mmol/L, K^+ 2.8 mmol/L, with alkalosis and normal renal function. Repeated tests confirmed the hypokalaemia. Estimation of plasma renin and aldosterone at 0800 h with the patient recumbent showed elevated aldosterone concentrations and suppressed renin activity, consistent with a diagnosis of primary hyperaldosteronism. An abdominal MRI scan was done that revealed a 4 cm mass in the left adrenal gland. Mr T was treated with spironolactone to control his blood pressure and correct the hypokalaemia and after 8 weeks his blood pressure was normalized and he underwent adrenal surgery and removal of a left-sided adrenal adenoma. Postoperatively, the spironolactone was withdrawn and his blood pressure remained within normal limits on no therapy.

Aldosterone

Aldosterone is the physiological mineralocorticoid of the body. In other words, it is an adrenal corticosteroid which affects cation concentrations and movements, specifically those of sodium (Na^+) and potassium (K^+).

Biosynthesis of aldosterone (Fig. 20a). Deoxycorticosterone (DOC), a weaker mineralocorticoid, is also secreted. Both are synthesized in the zona glomerulosa, which lacks the enzyme 17-hydoxylase. Progesterone is hydroxylated at C21 and C11-b, resulting in corticosterone, which is hydroxylated at C18 and then oxidized to an aldehyde. This is shown as the last reaction product in what is called the hemiacetal form and is the form in which it is predominantly present. The secretion of aldosterone is controlled by the renin–angiotensin system (Chapter 36) and, to a lesser extent, by ACTH. Essentially, hyperkalaemia (raised blood K^+), ACTH and angiotensin II can increase aldosterone release.

Mechanism of action of aldosterone (Fig. 20b). Aldosterone stimulates the active transport of sodium through the epithelial cell wall. In common with the other steroid hormones, aldosterone stimulates *de novo* synthesis of proteins, which enhance sodium transport in the epithelial cell of the distal convoluted tubule of the kidney, the site of aldosterone action in the nephron (Fig. 20c). The aldosterone receptor is also regulated by concentrations of aldosterone, higher concentrations of which reduce its production. Glucocorticoids bind to the aldosterone receptor with comparable affinity; furthermore, the same nuclear response element serves both glucocorticoid and aldosterone receptors. Nevertheless, glucocorticoids have only minor mineralocorticoid action because glucocorticoids are rapidly metabolized in cells that are principal targets for aldosterone. Conversely, aldosterone binds weakly to glucocorticoid receptors, explaining its glucocorticoid effect when administered in high doses. The drug **spironolactone** competes with aldosterone for its receptor.

There are three main theories to account for aldosterone action: (i) the hormone increases the number of sodium channels in the apical membrane; (ii) it increases the number of Na^+K^+-ATPase molecules; (iii) it increases adenosine triphosphate (ATP) molecule number within the cell. The hormone stimulates fatty acid synthesis and may alter membrane phospholipid composition as part of its mechanism of action.

Recent research suggests that aldosterone antagonists such as spironolactone may be useful for treatment of atrial fibrillation, given that aldosterone may be important in the aetiology of this cardiac disease.

The term **pseudohypoaldosteronism** encompasses rare genetic syndromescharacterized by hypertension and hypokalaemic alkalosis. Apparent mineralocorticoid excess (AME) is an autosomal dominant condition due to mutations in the gene encoding 11-β hydroxysteroid dehydrogenase Type II resulting in excessive glucocorticoid stimulation of mineralocorticoid receptors in the kidney. Liddle's syndrome is an autosomal dominant syndrome associated with abnormal functioning of epithelial Na channels causing sodium retention. AME is also mimicked by excess liquorice ingestion which blocks 11-β HSD.

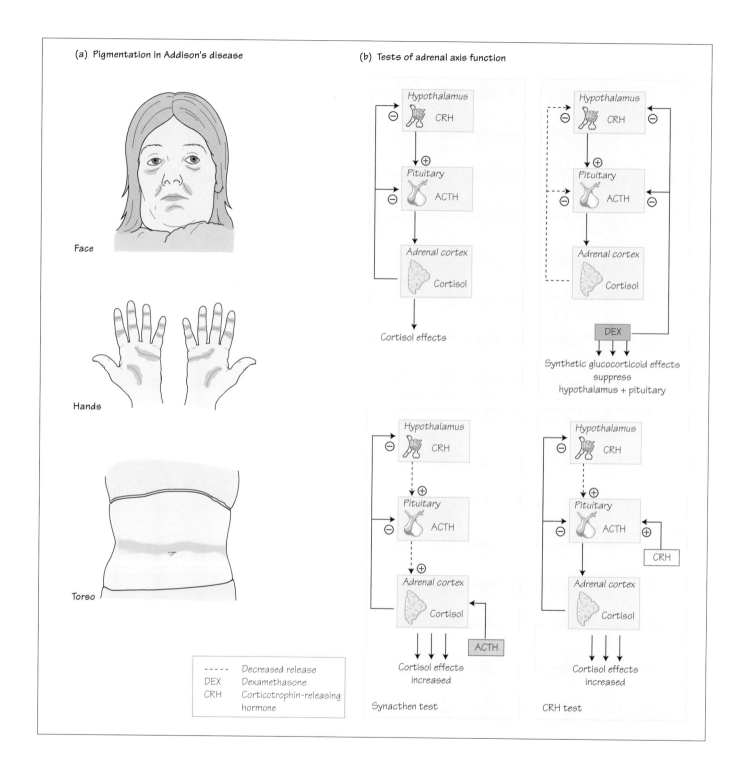

(a) Pigmentation in Addison's disease

Face

Hands

Torso

----- Decreased release
DEX   Dexamethasone
CRH   Corticotrophin-releasing hormone

(b) Tests of adrenal axis function

Hypothalamus
CRH
⊖
⊕
Pituitary
ACTH
⊖
Adrenal cortex
Cortisol
Cortisol effects

Hypothalamus
CRH
⊖   ⊖
⊕
Pituitary
ACTH
⊖
Adrenal cortex
Cortisol
DEX
Synthetic glucocorticoid effects
suppress
hypothalamus + pituitary

Hypothalamus
CRH
⊖
⊕
Pituitary
ACTH
⊖
⊕
Adrenal cortex
Cortisol
ACTH
Cortisol effects
increased
Synacthen test

Hypothalamus
CRH
⊖
⊕
Pituitary
ACTH
⊖   ⊕
CRH
Adrenal cortex
Cortisol
Cortisol effects
increased
CRH test

 The Endocrine System at a Glance, 3rd edition. © Ben Greenstein and Diana Wood. Published 2011 by Blackwell Publishing Ltd.

Clinical scenario

Adrenocortical insufficiency occurs as primary adrenal failure when the pathology lies in the adrenal gland, rather than secondary to failure of ACTH secretion. The symptoms may be vague, such as in the case of AD, a 22-year-old woman who presented with lethargy and fatigue. She was known to have autoimmune hypothyroidism and had been on thyroxine replacement therapy for 2 years. She now complained of increasing lethargy and intermittent abdominal pain. She became extremely unwell one day following an episode of food poisoning and was admitted to hospital as an emergency with diarrhoea, vomiting and hypotension. Examination revealed evidence of increased pigmentation of the palmar creases, over the knees and in the mouth, and hypotension with a postural fall in blood pressure of 30 mmHg. Blood tests showed her to have a blood sugar of 2.6 mmol/L, Na 131 mmol/L, K 5.6 mmol/ L and urea 12.6 mmol/L. A blood sample was saved for cortisol and ACTH estimation and she was treated with intravenous and subsequently oral hydrocortisone replacement therapy. Later results showed the plasma cortisol to be 95 nmol/L in combination with an ACTH concentration of 205 ng/L. A diagnosis of Addison's disease was made and she received advice from the endocrinology team about emergency hydrocortisone therapy, 'sick day rules' covering what to do in the event of intercurrent illness, and how to obtain a Medic-alert bracelet to wear continuously.

Adrenal hypofunction

Addison's disease. First described by Addison in 1855, the disease is caused by the destruction of adrenal tissue. The disease is usually autoimmune in origin, with the detection of adrenal autoantibodies in the plasma of 75–80% of patients, but there are numerous other causes (Table 21.1). The disease may present first as an Addisonian crisis, with fever, abdominal pain and hypotensive collapse and pigmentation of skin (Fig. 21a) and mucous membranes, due to very high circulating concentrations of adrenocorticotrophic hormone (ACTH). Areas often affected early include the skin under the fingernails, scars and buccal mucosa. The diagnosis is confirmed by measuring paired cortisol and ACTH (Fig. 21b). The presence of adrenal autantibodies is a helpful diagnostic indicator. There is hyperkalaemia, hyponatraemia, hypoglycaemia and high urine Na$^+$. Initial treatment, if the patient is in crisis, is intravenous saline solution to correct low blood volume, and hydrocortisone. Thereafter, the patient is maintained on oral glucocorticoids, for example **hydrocortisone** and the synthetic mineralocorticoid **fludrocortisone**.

Approximately 50% of patients with autoimmune Addison's disease have positive thyroid antibodies and/or other autoimmune endocrine phenomena (see Chapter 22).

Table 21.1 Causes of adrenal failure

Autoimmune	Alone or as part of a polyglandular autoimmune syndrome
Infection	TB
	Fungal infections
	HIV/AIDS
	Cytomegalovirus
Congenital	CAH
	Adrenal hypoplasia
	ACTH receptor gene mutations
	Triple A syndrome
	Adrenoleucodystrophy
	Adrenomyeloneuropathy
Drugs	Metyrapone[a]
	Ketoconazole[a]
	Aminoglutethamide[a]
	Barbiturates[b]
	Phenytoin[b]
	Rifampicin[b]
Others	Haemorrhage
	Metastatic tumour
	Amyloidosis
	Haemachromatosis
	Sarcoidosis
	Postadrenalectomy

[a] reduce cortisol synthesis.
[b] increase cortisol clearance.

In the Western world, autoimmune disease accounts for the majority of cases of adrenal insufficiency although worldwide tuberculosis, which causes infection and subsequent fibrosis of the adrenal glands, remains the most likely diagnosis. More recently, other infections such as cytomegalovirus and fungal infections are increasingly common in the context of HIV/AIDS. Malignant infiltration is also seen; the adrenals are a recognized site for metastatic spread from a number of malignancies and patients with AIDS may develop adrenal Kaposi's sarcoma.

Hypoaldosteronism, which is a deficiency of aldosterone release resulting in sodium loss, occurs in the following:

1 Addison's disease (see above) or specific enzyme deficiencies.

2 Diabetes, and may be secondary to deficient renin release. This may occur due to neuropathy which affects the β-adrenergic stimulation of renin release from the kidney.

3 Very rarely, some patients are insensitive to endogenous aldosterone because of an aldosterone receptor defect in the target cell.

22 Endocrine autoimmunity

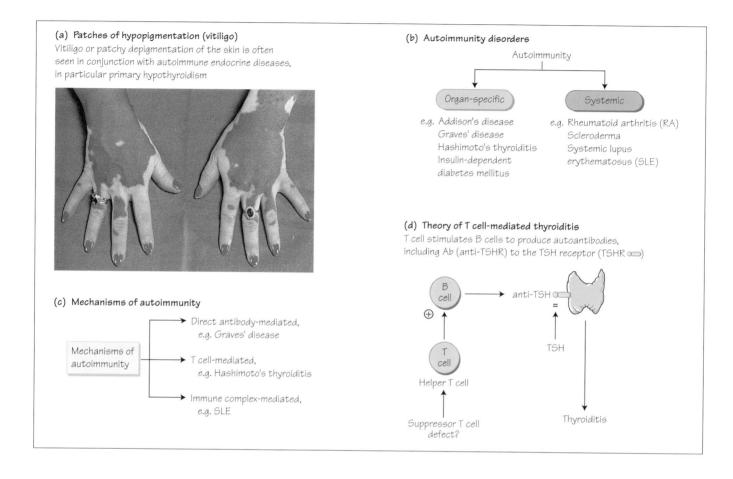

(a) Patches of hypopigmentation (vitiligo)
Vitiligo or patchy depigmentation of the skin is often seen in conjunction with autoimmune endocrine diseases, in particular primary hypothyroidism

(b) Autoimmunity disorders

Autoimmunity
- Organ-specific
  e.g. Addison's disease
       Graves' disease
       Hashimoto's thyroiditis
       Insulin-dependent
       diabetes mellitus
- Systemic
  e.g. Rheumatoid arthritis (RA)
       Scleroderma
       Systemic lupus
       erythematosus (SLE)

(c) Mechanisms of autoimmunity

Mechanisms of autoimmunity
- Direct antibody-mediated, e.g. Graves' disease
- T cell-mediated, e.g. Hashimoto's thyroiditis
- Immune complex-mediated, e.g. SLE

(d) Theory of T cell-mediated thyroiditis
T cell stimulates B cells to produce autoantibodies, including Ab (anti-TSHR) to the TSH receptor (TSHR)

B cell → anti-TSH
T cell (Helper T cell)
Suppressor T cell defect?
TSH
Thyroiditis

Clinical scenario

A 25-year-old woman, Mrs WG, was referred to the local endocrine clinic. She had visited her GP complaining of increasing tiredness and fatigue and, over the 4 weeks prior to presentation, had noticed she felt giddy at times, particularly when she got out of bed in the morning or on standing up from a chair. Mrs G was known to have primary hypothyroidism, on thyroxine replacement therapy and vitiligo over her forearms and chest. Her most recent set of thyroid function tests were in the normal range. The GP had noted her blood pressure to be 90/45. At the clinic the hypotension was confirmed and on questioning she had noticed increased pigmentation over her knees and around her waistband. A short Synacthen test was performed during which her basal plasma cortisol level was found to be 75 nmol/L and 100 nmol/L 30 minutes after injection of 250 μg of synthetic ACTH (Synacthen). Later her basal ACTH concentration was reported at 550 ng/L and adrenal antibodies were positive, confirming the diagnosis of primary adrenal failure. She was started on glucocorticoid replacement in the form of hydrocortisone and mineralocorticoid replacement with fludrocortisone, following which her symptoms rapidly improved.

Many endocrine conditions have an autoimmune aetiology and patients frequently exhibit antibodies to multiple endocrine organs and have evidence of associated autoimmune disease such as pernicious anaemia, depigmentation of the skin (vitiligo; Fig. 22a) or coeliac disease. Two specific autoimmune polyglandular syndromes are recognized in which there are two or more affected endocrine glands as well as non-endocrine manifestations (Table 22.1):
- PGA 1 presents in children and is an autoimmune recessive disorder;
- PGA 2 (also known as Schmidt's syndrome) is a familial disorder most commonly seen in women and thought to be HLA DR3 linked.

Autoimmunity

Autoimmunity may be defined as an attack by the host's immune system on the host's own tissues. These attacks may be transient immune reactions to infection, for example, which resolve spontaneously. They may, however, become chronic, with pathological consequences. Endocrine autoimmunity often involves an immune attack on specific endocrine glands, for

Table 22.1 Polyglandular autoimmune syndromes (adapted from J O'Connell and D O'Shea, Addison's disease, in: S Robinson and K Meeran (eds), *Endocrinology Specialist Handbook*, Martin Dunitz, London, 2002)

PGA 1	Prevalence of disorder (%)	PGA 2	Prevalence of disorder (%)
Hypoparathyroidism	93	Adrenal failure	100
Mucocutaneous candidiasis	83	Autoimmune thyroid disease	70
Adrenal failure	73	Type 1 diabetes	50
Hypogonadism	43	Primary gonadal failure	5–50
Coeliac disease	15		
Pernicious anaemia	15	Vitiligo	4
Thyroid disease	10		
Chronic active hepatitis	20		
Vitiligo	15		
Type 1 diabetes	2		

example Addison's disease, Graves' disease, Hashimoto's thyroiditis and insulin-dependent diabetes mellitus, where the gland is damaged or destroyed altogether. These are examples of mainly **organ-specific** autoimmune diseases (Fig. 22b). In **systemic** autoimmune disease, on the other hand, the immune system attacks several tissues that may be anatomically distant from each other. Examples of systemic autoimmune disease include rheumatoid arthritis, scleroderma and systemic lupus erythematosus (SLE). There may be both organ-specific and systemic components in most, if not all, autoimmune diseases. Some autoimmune diseases may have genetic and/or endocrine components, since some, notably Graves' disease (thyrotoxicosis), Hashimoto's thyroiditis, rheumatoid arthritis (RA) and SLE, are more prevalent in women, and the sex hormones, especially estrogens, may be important mediating factors.

Mechanisms of autoimmunity. These are not well understood at the moment, but three important mechanisms have been defined so far: (i) direct antibody-mediated; (ii) T cell-mediated; and (iii) immune complex-mediated (Fig. 22c). While autoimmune diseases might tentatively be classified in terms of these three mechanisms, it is possible that all three are involved in an autoimmune disease.

1 Direct antibody-mediated disease: Graves' disease is an example of direct antibody action on a gland causing damage. The disease can be passively transferred from a diseased to a healthy organism by the transfer of IgG antibodies. For example, babies born of mothers who have untreated Graves' disease exhibit symptoms of thyroiditis until the baby's system destroys the IgG which had been transferred via the placenta. In severe cases, the baby may be successfully treated using plasma exchange.

2 T cell-mediated disease: Hashimoto's thyroiditis is an example of this type of endocrine autoimmunity (Fig. 22d). In these patients, autoreactive T cells cause tissue damage in the thyroid by two main mechanisms: (i) they recruit and activate macrophages, which destroy tissues; and (ii) T cells release cytokines, for example tissue necrosis factor (TNF). Possibly, suppressor T-cell function is impaired in these patients, and helper T cells inappropriately stimulate autoantibody production in B cell, including the production of TSH receptor antibodies, which bind to the TSH receptor on thyrocytes. In addition

to these T cell-mediated effects, iodine uptake and thyroglobulin binding may be directly interfered with by autoreactive antibodies. Furthermore, the inflammation caused by autoimmune reactions may trigger apoptosis in thyrocytes. Thyrocytes, unusually, constitutively express the FAS receptor ligand, which combines with the FAS receptor to cause apoptosis of the thyrocytes.

3 Immune complex-mediated disease: systemic autoimmune diseases, such as SLE, are most probably caused by immune complex-mediated reactions. Patients with SLE have several circulating autoantibodies to both cytoplasmic and nuclear constituents, for example IgG directed against double-stranded nuclear DNA. The cytoplasmic and nuclear antigens may not themselves be pathogenic; a major pathogenic event is the deposition of the immune complexes in tissues such as the kidneys.

Genetic factors. Epidemiological and familial studies of virtually all autoimmune diseases point to a genetic susceptibility. The most important genetic determinant appears to be the major histocompatibility complex (MHC), a series of genes on chromosome 6 that code for antigens, including the human leukocyte antigen (HLA) system. Recent research suggests that there are multiple genetic loci that contribute to autoimmune diseases such as insulin-dependent diabetes mellitus (IDDM). In the case of IDDM, the gene encoding preproinsulin may be a locus for genetic polymorphism that may be associated with susceptibility to IDDM.

Endocrine factors. The possible role of endocrine hormones, for example estrogens, in the aetiology of autoimmune disease is unknown at present, but the sexual dimorphism of the distribution of several autoimmune diseases points to the involvement of the sex hormones. This putative role for sex hormones is given support from the well-known phenomenon of RA remission during pregnancy, and the rebound exacerbation or 'flare' of disease after parturition. SLE, as mentioned above, is far more common in women, especially during the reproductive years, and often flares up during pregnancy and after parturition. SLE may be precipitated or flare after commencement of oral contraceptive use. It has been reported that patients with SLE and their first-degree relatives had elevated serum levels of 16α-hydroxyestrone, which is an actively feminizing metabolite of estradiol.

23 Sexual differentiation and development: I Introduction

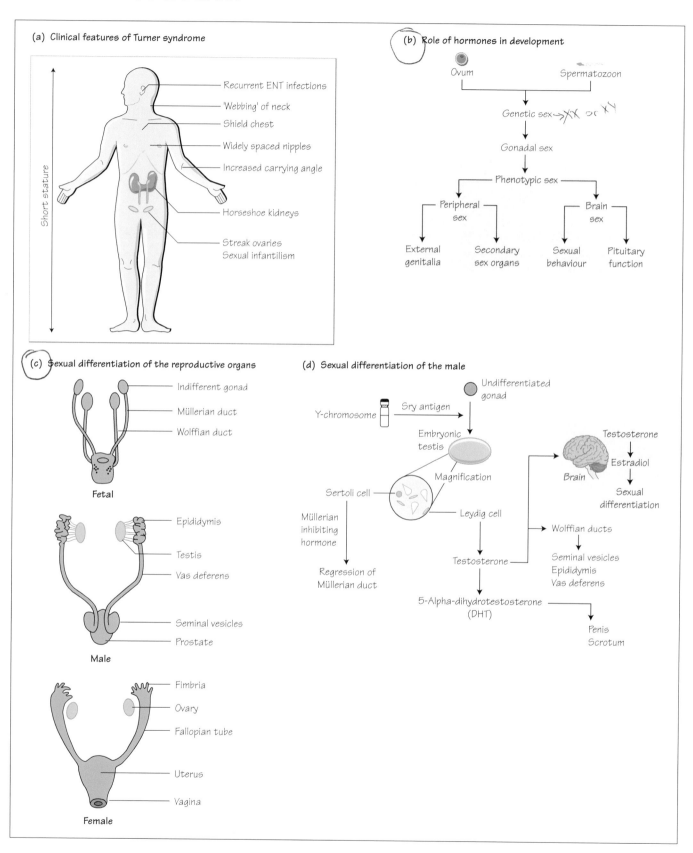

(a) Clinical features of Turner syndrome

- Recurrent ENT infections
- 'Webbing' of neck
- Shield chest
- Widely spaced nipples
- Increased carrying angle
- Horseshoe kidneys
- Streak ovaries Sexual infantilism

Short stature

(b) Role of hormones in development

Ovum   Spermatozoon

Genetic sex → XX or XY

Gonadal sex

Phenotypic sex

Peripheral sex

- External genitalia
- Secondary sex organs

Brain sex

- Sexual behaviour
- Pituitary function

(c) Sexual differentiation of the reproductive organs

- Indifferent gonad
- Müllerian duct
- Wolffian duct

Fetal

- Epididymis
- Testis
- Vas deferens
- Seminal vesicles
- Prostate

Male

- Fimbria
- Ovary
- Fallopian tube
- Uterus
- Vagina

Female

(d) Sexual differentiation of the male

Undifferentiated gonad

Y-chromosome → Sry antigen → Embryonic testis

Magnification

Sertoli cell   Leydig cell

Müllerian inhibiting hormone → Regression of Müllerian duct

Testosterone

5-Alpha-dihydrotestosterone (DHT)

Brain → Testosterone → Estradiol → Sexual differentiation

Wolffian ducts

- Seminal vesicles
- Epididymis
- Vas deferens

Penis Scrotum

Clinical scenario

Miss JP was referred to the paediatric endocrine clinic at the age of 14 years because her periods had not started and she was noted to be of short stature. On examination in the clinic she was found to be below the 3rd centile of height for her age. She had a number of dysmorphic features including a 'webbed' appearance to her neck, a wide carrying angle of the arms and widely spaced nipples with absent breast development (Fig. 23a). Turner syndrome was confirmed by the findings of raised gonadotrophin concentrations in the presence of an abnormal karyotype, 45XO. She was treated with low-dose ethinylestradiol and growth hormone to maximize growth, with subsequent increasing doses of estradiol to initiate pubertal development, followed by combined estrogen/ progestogens to maintain a menstrual cycle.

Genetic sex

Sexual differentiation can be classified according to: (i) the genetic sex of the phenotype, that is whether it is XX or XY with respect to the sex chromosomes; and (ii) according to the sexual characteristics determined by the gonadal hormones (Fig. 23b). Every human normally has 46 chromosomes in each cell, consisting of 22 pairs of autosomal chromosomes, and a pair of sex chromosomes. Genetic sex is determined at the time of conception, when male and female gametes fuse to form a new individual. The possession of a Y chromosome determines that a male will develop, as the Y chromosome possesses the sex-determining gene, also called the Sry gene, which expresses the Sry antigen. The Sry antigen is a trigger that switches on genes on other chromosomes responsible for testicular development.

Gonadal sex

In the human fetus, at about 4 weeks, the gonads are indifferent, that is they cannot be distinguished as testis or ovary, and are capable of developing into either (Fig. 23c). The indifferent gonad before differentiation is composed of a coating of germinal epithelium, the genital ridge mesenchyme and the primordial germ cells. Thereafter, under the influence of the Sry antigen (Fig. 23d), the primordial germ cells will move to what is called the medullary region of the primitive gonad. Still under Sry influence, the indifferent gonad begins to develop into a testis. Primitive sex cords give rise to the seminiferous tubules, whose lining of epithelial cells will differentiate into the germinal epithelium, which will give rise to the spermatogonia and the Sertoli cells. These epithelial cells also differentiate into the Leydig cells, which will produce the male sex hormone testosterone. Where the seminiferous tubule leaves the testis, it branches extensively to form the rete testis, which transports the sperm to the tubules. In the absence of the Sry antigen, the ovary develops. The ovary develops later than does the testis, although both gonadal forms develop steroidogenic competence at the same time.

Phenotypic sex: secondary sexual characteristics

Ductal differentiation. Before differentiation, the ductal systems are bipotential. If a testis develops, it produces a Müllerian inhibiting hormone, also known as anti-Müllerian hormone (AMH). AMH is a glycoprotein of molecular weight about 70 kDa, which causes atrophy of the Müllerian ducts. The testis Leydig cells also start to secrete testosterone, which supports the development of the Wolffian ducts. This, in turn, leads to the development of the epididymis, seminal vesicles and the ductus deferens. In the absence of the ovaries and testis (i.e. if they are removed from the developing fetus or not functioning), the Müllerian ducts develop and the Wolffian ducts wither, which suggests that the gonads are not required for the development of a female ductal system.

External genitalia. In the absence of the Y chromosome, the female phenotypical external genitalia will develop. When the fetal testis starts producing androgen, the penis and scrotum form and the testes descend. In the female, the genital tubercle will become the clitoris and the labia will develop.

With the exception of Turner syndrome, syndromes of gonadal dysgenesis are rare. Girls with gonadal dysgenesis usually present with failure of pubertal development and primary amenorrhoea. Abnormalities of the X chromosome, such as partial deletions, multiplication and structural rearrangements, may present with primary or secondary amenorrhoea and absent or delayed puberty, possibly with some of the somatic abnormalities seen in Turner syndrome. Rarely, girls presenting with delayed puberty are found to have 46XX pure gonadal dysgenesis (associated with undetectable ovarian tissue) or to have the 46XY karyoptype. In the latter case, early failure of testicular development results in inactive gonads and feminization of the internal and external genitalia. Patients with gonadal dysgenesis in association with a Y chromosome have a high risk of developing gonadal tumours in testicular remnants and surgery is recommended to remove any intra-abdominal testicular tissue.

Klinefelter's syndrome in males is characterized by a range of abnormal clinical features, from degrees of feminization to normal male habitus. Karyotypes vary from XXY, XXYY, XXXY to mosaic forms, usually XY/XXY. There is dysgenesis of the seminiferous tubules resulting in small, firm testes and absent spermatogenesis (although rarely spermatogenesis and even fertility may be present in mosaic individuals). Most patients with Klinefelter's syndrome are tall, infertile and have gynaecomastia.

Classical Turner syndrome associated with a 45XO karyotype is the commonest form of gonadal dysgenesis. The ovaries are present only as fibrous 'streaks' resulting in pubertal failure and primary amenorrhoea. Short stature is always present and may respond to growth hormone (GH) therapy although higher doses of GH are required than needed in children with isolated GH deficiency and there is thought to be a degree of skeletal dysplasia causing end-organ resistance to treatment. There is a wide individual response to GH in girls with Turner syndrome, although most show some improvement with treatment. A number of clinical features may be present, as in Fig. 23a, as well as various other abnormalities, particularly of the renal tract and otolaryngeal system. Induction of puberty with low-dose ethinyl estradiol is associated with breast development and growth and maturation of the genital tract. Subsequent combined estrogen/ progestogen treatment results in maintenance of the menstrual cycle and prevention of osteoporosis. Other patients have mosaic karyotypes (usually 45XO/ 46XX) and may have few physical signs other than primary amenorrhoea. Rarely, such patients menstruate for some years and may present with secondary amenorrhoea.

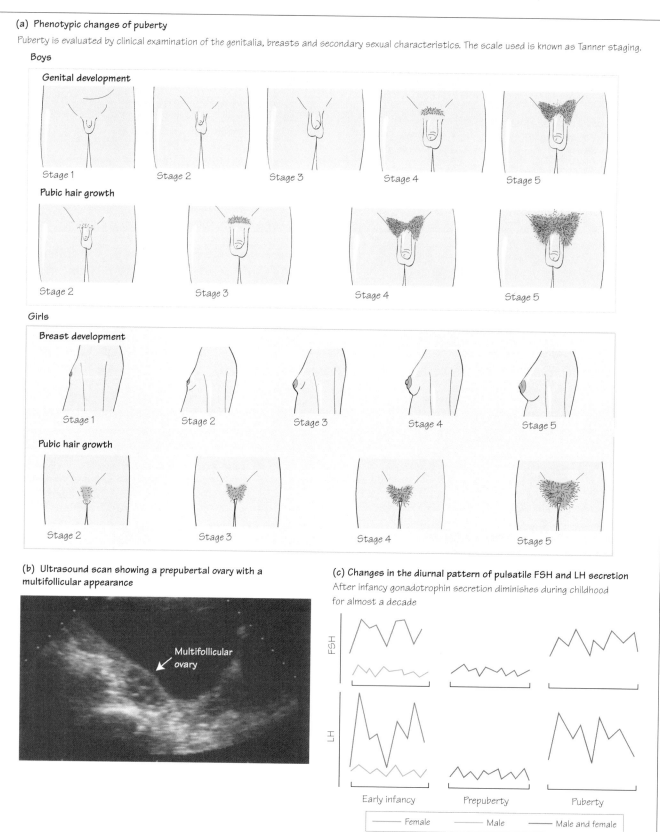

(a) Phenotypic changes of puberty

Puberty is evaluated by clinical examination of the genitalia, breasts and secondary sexual characteristics. The scale used is known as Tanner staging.

Boys

Genital development

Stage 1 Stage 2 Stage 3 Stage 4 Stage 5

Pubic hair growth

Stage 2 Stage 3 Stage 4 Stage 5

Girls

Breast development

Stage 1 Stage 2 Stage 3 Stage 4 Stage 5

Pubic hair growth

Stage 2 Stage 3 Stage 4 Stage 5

(b) Ultrasound scan showing a prepubertal ovary with a multifollicular appearance

Multifollicular ovary

(c) Changes in the diurnal pattern of pulsatile FSH and LH secretion

After infancy gonadotrophin secretion diminishes during childhood for almost a decade

FSH

LH

Early infancy Prepuberty Puberty

Female —— Male —— Male and female ——

Clinical background

Delayed puberty is one of the most common referrals to paediatric and adult endocrine clinics. It is defined as absence of breast development in a girl by 13.5 years or failure of testicular growth to >4 ml by 14 years in a boy. Constitutional delay of puberty is by far the most common diagnosis in boys, accounting for around 80% of cases, whereas in girls delayed puberty is more likely to reflect serious underlying pathology. Clinical assessment of boys with delayed puberty should be aimed towards identifying patients with individual underlying pathology. If constitutional delay is confirmed then treatment is conservative to observe any spontaneous development over 6–8 months. If no pubertal change is evident then treatment with low-dose testosterone will induce hypothalamic–pituitary activity and trigger the onset of puberty. In girls with delayed puberty and primary amenorrhoea a specific cause is more usually found. Clinical examination will establish signs of Turner syndrome and subsequent investigations must include karyotype analysis. Treatment is specific for the underlying cause.

Puberty

Puberty describes a series of events associated with a growth spurt and culminating in the acquisition of sexual maturity and reproductive function. The phenotypic changes of puberty follow a set pattern (Fig. 24a). Any deviation from the 'consonance' of puberty suggests an underlying abnormality. The timing of puberty is influenced by genetic factors and, critically, by body weight and composition. Over the last century, in the Western world, the age of onset of puberty has become earlier, in association with an increase in final height. In boys, puberty begins with the attainment of testicular volumes of 4 ml but the growth spurt occurs late in puberty and is predicted by a testicular volume of 10 ml. Conversely, in girls growth is an early pubertal event occurring with the onset of breast development.

Growth and puberty. Increases in gonadal steroid production at puberty stimulate the production of growth hormone. GH is secreted in a pulsatile fashion at night and there is an increase in the amplitude of GH pulses during normal puberty, although not their frequency. Increased GH secretion is reflected in the pubertal growth spurt which forms a crucial part of the maturational processes during adolescence. Absence or delay in the growth spurt usually indicates lack of consonance of puberty and requires investigation.

Adrenarche. Adrenal androgen secretion increases before puberty, at about age 6–8 years, and is associated with the onset of the development of axillary and pubic hair and apocrine sweat glands and, usually, a small increase in height velocity.

Endocrine regulation of puberty

The hypothalamic–pituitary–gonadal axis is active in fetal life with high gonadotrophin concentrations seen in the first half of gestation followed by reduced levels in the second half, thought to be due to a developing negative feedback system by gonadal steroids. In the immediate postnatal period gonadotrophin levels are high, related to the withdrawal of placental steroids and alterations to the negative feedback equilibrium. Gonadotrophin levels subsequently fall and remain low throughout early childhood, although detectable LH pulses can be identified as early as 6 years.

The onset of puberty is marked by a rise in LH secretion, which occurs firstly as nocturnal pulses. This occurs several years before the onset of phenotypic puberty and is in response to increased GnRH secretion and enhanced responsiveness of the pituitary gonadotrophs to the GnRH stimulus. Evidence for pulsatile LH secretion can be seen in ovarian ultrasound scans of normal prepubertal girls which show multiple ovarian follicles distributed throughout the ovary, an appearance typical of pulsatile LH input (Fig. 24b).

The factors that regulate the onset of LH secretion at the start of puberty remain to be fully elucidated but a number of neurotransmitters and other endocrine, paracrine and autocrine factors have been identified that modify the hypothalamic–pituitary–gonadal axis at this time. It has been recognized for some time that body weight and body composition affect the onset of puberty and the hormone leptin, derived from peripheral adipose tissue, plays a major role in signalling changes in body composition to the hypothalamus.

LH secretion gradually increases with the establishment of regular LH pulses occurring every 90 minutes during both night and day. LH secretion results in the production of gonadal steroids and the onset of secondary sexual characteristics. Increasing gonadal steroid concentrations regulate the GnRH pulse generator, establishing the mature diurnal variation and feedback systems seen in both sexes. In girls, estrogen levels rise dramatically in the year before menarche, establishing the positive feedback needed to induce a preovulatory LH surge. In boys, the regular LH pulses result in peak testosterone concentrations in the early mornings (Fig. 24c).

Gonadal development in childhood and puberty

In males, there is a rise in testosterone production between the ages of 2 and 4 months associated with Leydig cell multiplication but after that the testes remain relatively inactive until the onset of puberty. Testicular size increases from around the age of 10 years, reflecting increased gonadotrophin secretion and growth of seminiferous tubules.

In females, the elevated gonadotrophin levels seen after birth decline by the age of 2–3 years and remain low throughout childhood. The rise in gonadotrophin secretion seen by the age of 6 is associated with the development of antral follicles in the ovary and a rise in estrogen concentration. The commencement of sex hormone production and release during puberty is accompanied by gonadal and accessory sex organ growth and function. The end of puberty is marked by the menarche with the onset of regular ovulatory cycles.

25 Female reproduction: I Menstrual cycle

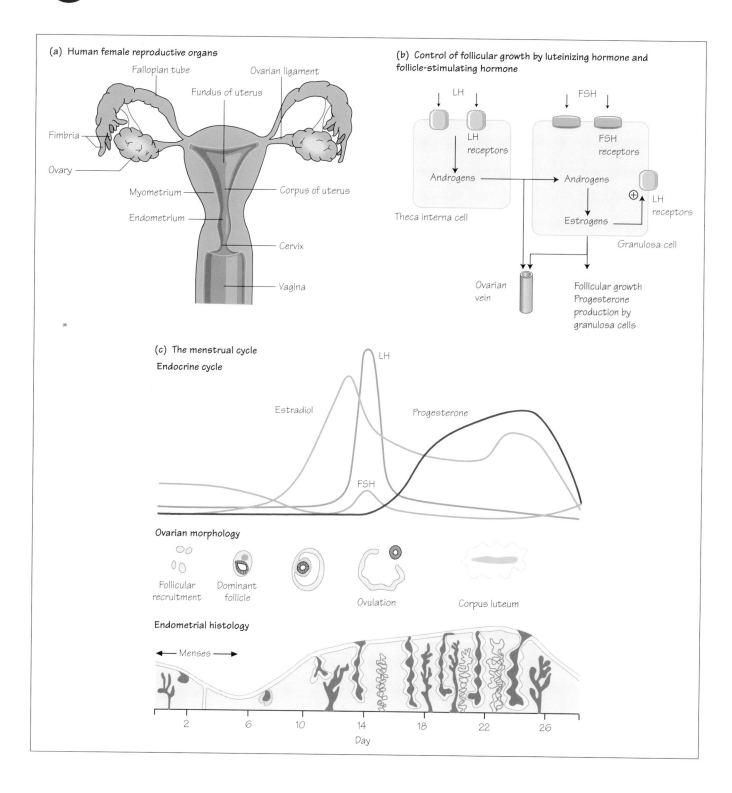

(a) Human female reproductive organs

(b) Control of follicular growth by luteinizing hormone and follicle-stimulating hormone

(c) The menstrual cycle

Endocrine cycle

Ovarian morphology

Endometrial histology

Clinical background

The end of puberty in females is associated with the onset of regular ovulatory menstrual cycles. The menstrual cycle represents complex hormonal changes involving the ovaries, hypothalamus and pituitary and is characterized by ovarian follicular maturation, ovulation of a dominant follicle and formation of a corpus luteum. The first day of bleeding is day 1 of the cycle and marks the onset of the follicular phase which culminates in the LH surge (day 12–14), ovulation and the onset of the luteal phase. During the luteal phase progesterone is secreted by the corpus luteum causing characteristic changes in the endometrium. In the absence of pregnancy, endometrial changes regress at the end of the luteal phase causing breakdown and the onset of bleeding. In normal women, the menstrual cycle lasts 28 days although this may be less regular at either end of the reproductive years.

Clinically, monitoring of the menstrual cycle may be useful in the assessment of subfertility. Monitoring of cycle dates should be performed, including other symptoms such as mid-cycle lower abdominal pain and increased cervical secretion. Progesterone secretion causes basal body temperature to rise in the second half of the cycle and early morning temperature rises of 0.5°C indicate the onset of the luteal phase. In the assessment of ovulatory disorders ultrasound scanning may be used to track follicular development and elevation of the serum progesterone concentration on day 21 of the cycle confirms ovulation.

Female reproductive organs

The female reproductive organs are the ovaries, the fallopian tubes, the uterus and the vagina (Fig. 25a). The ovaries produce the estrogens, progesterone and the ovum. After ovulation, the ovum is released into the abdominal cavity, where it is swept up by the fimbriae of the oviducts, and passes into the fallopian tube. Here it may be fertilized, and the fertilized ovum, or morula, passes into the uterus, where it is implanted into the uterine endometrium and grows to become the fetus. Usually, a single ovum is released each cycle from the human ovary.

The menstrual cycle

The principal functions of the female reproductive system are to produce the ovum and to ensure that it is fertilized, nurtured and allowed to grow, and to expel it safely into the external environment. The production of the ovum depends upon the orchestration of a number of hormone-dependent events which culminate in ovulation (Fig. 25b). Inside the ovary during each cycle, many follicles or groups of cells are developing, but only one will de-velop fully and the others will undergo atresia (degeneration). The follicle develops under the influence of luteinizing hor-mone (LH), which stimulates estrogen produc-tion, and follicle-stimulating hormone, (FSH) which promotes follicular growth and induces LH receptors (Fig. 25c). The ovarian granulosa cells produce a protein hormone, inhibin, which is able to suppress FSH secretion from the pituitary. It has been found that subunits of inhibin can actually stimulate the release of FSH, and so the protein may have a complex but important role in the regulation of follicular maturation.

Estrogen is produced by the ovary during follicular maturation, and stimulates glandular proliferation of the inner lining or endometrium of the uterus – the proliferative phase. At the same time, the hormone stimulates the synthesis of progesterone receptors, thus preparing the uterus for subsequent large concentrations of progesterone. This hormone makes the endometrium secretory, in preparation for the fertilized ovum. The vagina, too, alters cyclically. As estrogen rises, so the vaginal epithelium proliferates. If fertilization does not occur, then towards the end of the luteal phase the epithelium is invaded by leukocytes and cast off by the underlying epithelium, representing new growth at the beginning of the next cycle.

The characteristics of the cervical mucus are dependent on the hormonal milieu. During the follicular phase, the mucus is watery, but progesterone changes the mucus to a more viscous form, with minute channels through which the spermatozoa pass on their way to the ovum.

During the preovulatory or follicular phase of the cycle, circulating FSH is low, but as estrogen and inhibin concentrations rise, they continue feed back to suppress FSH release. Negative feedback of estrogen keeps LH release low, as in the early follicular phase. However, rising estrogen concentrations towards the end of the follicular phase sensitize the pituitary gonadotrophs to GnRH, resulting in the massive preovulatory LH surge and the triggering of ovulation.

At maturation, the follicle, which is now termed a Graafian follicle, produces less estrogen and more progesterone, and these hormones appear to act in concert to produce, together with GnRH, a massive release of LH into the bloodstream. The LH causes the follicle to rupture, and the ovum is released. The follicle now becomes the progesterone-secreting corpus luteum and the postovulatory period is termed the luteal phase of the menstrual cycle. If fertilization does not occur, the corpus luteum gradually releases less and less progesterone as it runs its limited lifespan and becomes the corpus albicans (white body). The spiral arteries shrivel, the endometrium collapses due to a lack of blood, and the lining is lost with the menstrual flow. The events described above are termed the menstrual cycle, and occur approximately monthly for the reproductive life of women.

The menstrual cycle varies with the individual, but is taken on average as 28 days, and is numbered from the first day of vaginal bleeding or menses.

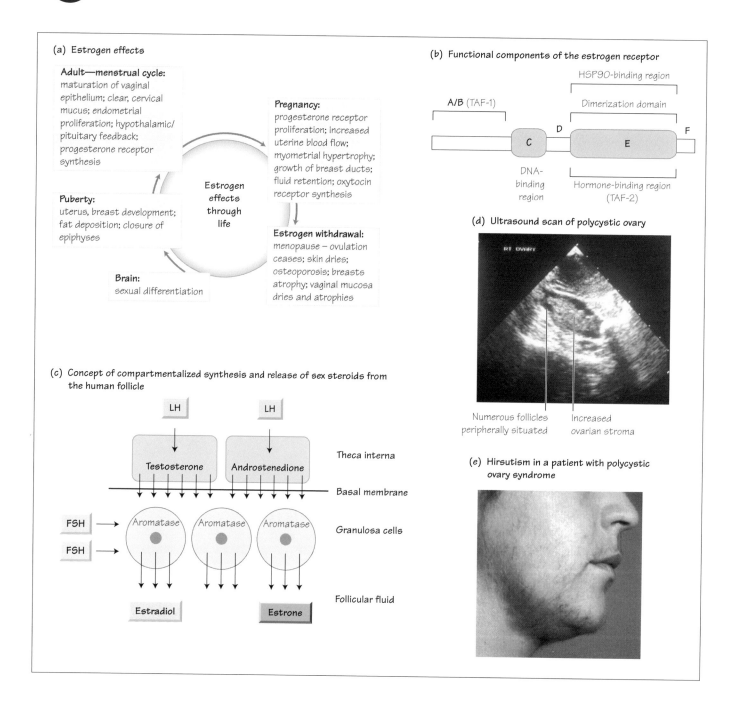

(a) Estrogen effects

Adult—menstrual cycle: maturation of vaginal epithelium; clear, cervical mucus; endometrial proliferation; hypothalamic/pituitary feedback; progesterone receptor synthesis

Pregnancy: progesterone receptor proliferation; increased uterine blood flow; myometrial hypertrophy; growth of breast ducts; fluid retention; oxytocin receptor synthesis

Puberty: uterus, breast development; fat deposition; closure of epiphyses

Estrogen effects through life

Estrogen withdrawal: menopause – ovulation ceases; skin dries; osteoporosis; breasts atrophy; vaginal mucosa dries and atrophies

Brain: sexual differentiation

(b) Functional components of the estrogen receptor

HSP90-binding region

A/B (TAF-1)

Dimerization domain

C   D   E   F

DNA-binding region

Hormone-binding region (TAF-2)

(d) Ultrasound scan of polycystic ovary

RT OVARY

Numerous follicles peripherally situated   Increased ovarian stroma

(c) Concept of compartmentalized synthesis and release of sex steroids from the human follicle

LH   LH

Testosterone   Androstenedione   Theca interna

Basal membrane

FSH   Aromatase   Aromatase   Aromatase   Granulosa cells

FSH

Estradiol   Estrone   Follicular fluid

(e) Hirsutism in a patient with polycystic ovary syndrome

Clinical scenario

Miss RB, a 24-year-old woman, presented to her GP complaining of increasing hair growth over her chin and face with greasy skin and acne. The hair growth had been present for 5 or 6 years but over the last 2 years had become much worse, such that she was shaving her chin three times a week and using a number of depilatory creams purchased at the chemists. On questioning she revealed that she had also noticed increased hair growth around her nipples, over her lower abdomen and on the lower part of her back. Her periods started when she was 12 years old but she had never had a regular cycle; her periods only occurred every 6–10 weeks and on one occasion she had missed her period for 4 months. She had always been 'overweight' but had gained 2 stones in weight over the last 2 years. Her mother had had irregular menses and had been treated for subfertility prior to conceiving RB. Her maternal grandmother had Type 2 diabetes mellitus. On examination RB was found to be obese with a body mass index of 32 kg/m². She had marked androgen-dependent hirsutism and a Ferriman and Galwey score was found to be 16. The diagnosis of polycystic ovary syndrome was confirmed when subsequent biochemical investigations showed her to have a raised testosterone concentration of 3.2 nmol/L, LH 14.5 U/L, FSH 3.3 U/L and an ultrasound scan of the ovaries showed bilaterally enlarged ovaries with numerous peripherally sited follicles. After discussion she was treated with diet, exercise and the drug metformin, all of which lower insulin resistance and reduce ovarian androgen secretion. This combination resulted in improvement in the hirsutism and establishment of a more regular menstrual cycle.

Polycystic ovary syndrome is the commonest cause of hirsutism and irregular menstrual cycles. Patients have a long history, usually dating back to the menarche. It is important in the assessment of women with hirsutism to exclude those with a short history and features of virilization that might suggest androgen-secreting tumours of the ovary or adrenal glands.

Physiological actions of estrogens

The effects of the estrogens can be classified in chronological order of the major reproductive events of the female (Fig. 26a). Overall, their main influence is on the maintenance of fertility.

Sexual differentiation. During fetal development, estrogens are not required for the normal differentiation and development of the female genitalia and accessory sex organs, but they are needed for sexual differentiation of the brain.

Puberty. During puberty (see Chapter 24), estrogens stimulate development of the breast stroma, endometrium, myometrium and vagina. Estrogens cause epiphyseal closure and characteristic fat deposition in peripheral tissues.

Adult. In the adult female, estrogens maintain the menstrual cycle and female secondary sexual characteristics. Estrogens facilitate the actions of progesterone by stimulating the synthesis of progesterone receptors, notably in the brain and uterus.

Pregnancy. During pregnancy, estrogens increase the blood flow to and through the uterus, they cause hypertrophy of the uterine myometrium and stimulate breast ductal proliferation. They enhance fluid retention and stimulate uterine progesterone receptor synthesis. Shortly before parturition (birth), estrogens stimulate the synthesis of oxytocin receptors in the uterus myometrium. Oxytocin is involved in parturition through its contractile action on the uterus (see Chapter 34).

Metabolic effects. Estrogen inhibits bone resorption, an action which becomes apparent after the menopause, when estrogen wanes. Estrogens decrease bowel motility. They affect liver function by stimulating protein synthesis, including that of sex hormone-binding globulin (SHBG) and thyroxine-binding globulin (see 13). Estrogens affect blood coagulability by stimulating the production of factors II, VII, IX, and X but decreasing platelet aggregation. They have important effects on plasma lipids, decreasing total cholesterol, increasing high-density lipoprotein (HDL) and decreasing low-density lipoprotein (LDL) concentrations.

Menopause marks the cessation of natural female reproductive life. The ovaries no longer produce ova, and the secretion of estrogens declines and eventually ceases. The symptoms associated with the menopause vary from individual to individual

and between cultural groups. Vasomotor instability causing hot flushes and sweating, vaginal dryness and an increased rate of bone resorption, potentially leading to osteopaenia and osteoporosis, are the only established features of estrogen deficiency and are relieved by estrogen replacement therapy.

Mechanism of action of estrogens

Estrogens travel in the bloodstream, largely bound to plasma proteins, and diffuse into the cell and the nucleus where they bind to specific receptor proteins (Chapter 4).

Two main forms of the estrogen receptor have been discovered, namely ER-α and ER-β. ER-α is the form that dictates much of sexual function and behaviour, and may be the form of the receptor responsible for breast and other estrogen-mediated cancers. There is evidence that the ratio of ER-α: ER-β is an important determinant of health and disease, especially with regard to carcinogenicity of estrogen. The estrogen receptor proteins have been characterized and have different multifunctional domains (Fig. 26b). The receptor has at least two transcriptional activation functional sites (TAF-1 and 2; see also Chapter 4), a DNA-binding domain, which is similar for many of the DNA-binding receptors, and a hormone-specific binding domain.

Ovarian androgens

The ovary is also an important source of androgen production in the female, accounting for about 50% (the rest being adrenal in origin). Androstenedione and testosterone are synthesized in the theca cell layer of the maturing follicle under the influence of LH. They diffuse into granulosa cells where they are aromatized to form estrogens (Fig. 26c). Androgens and the other steroid and peptide hormones produced in the developing follicle are important local regulators of ovarian function and folliculogenesis. In mature females, many of the common disorders of reproductive function are associated with excessive androgen production, disordered folliculogenesis and ovulation and subsequent subfertility associated with the peripheral effects of excess androgen production (Figs 26d and e).

Table 26.1 The Ferriman–Gallwey hirsutism grading system (condensed)

	Site	Definitions
1	Upper lip	1: a few hairs at outer margins, to 4: a moustache extending to midline
2	Chin	1: a few scattered hairs, to 4: complete heavy cover
3	Chest	1: circumareolar hairs, to 4: complete cover
4	Upper back	1: a few scattered hairs, to 4: complete heavy cover
5	Lower back	1: a sacral tuft of hair, to 4: complete cover
6	Upper abdomen	1: a few midline hairs, to 4: complete cover
7	Lower abdomen	1: a few midline hairs, to 4: an inverted V-shaped growth
8	Arm	1: sparse growth < one-quarter of limb surface, to 4: complete heavy growth
9	Forearm	Complete cover of dorsal surface; 1: very light to 4: very heavy
10	Thigh	As for arm
11	Leg	As for arm

27 Female reproduction: III Pregnancy

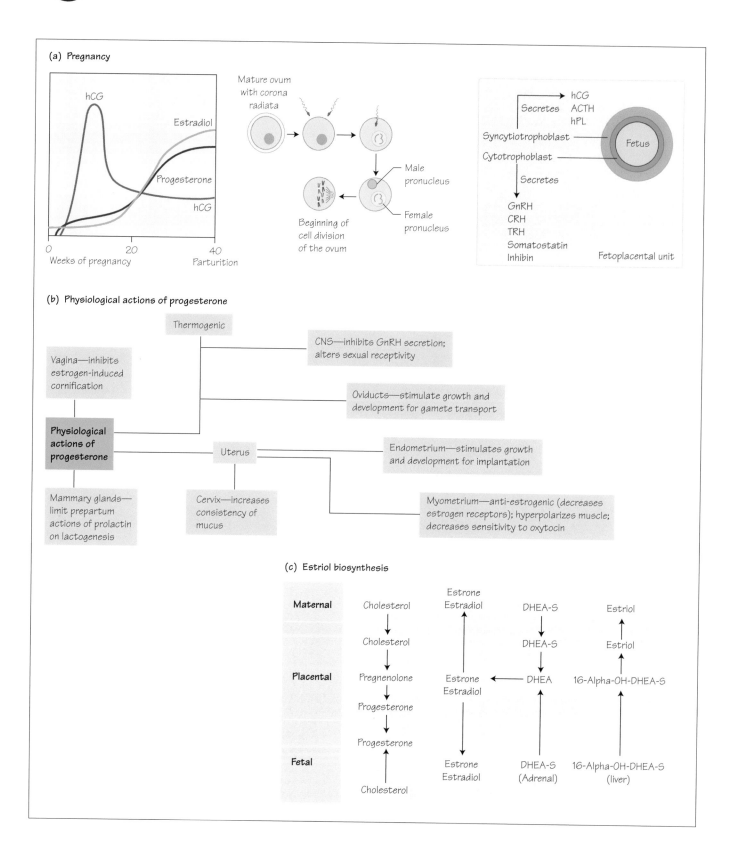

(a) Pregnancy

hCG
Estradiol
Progesterone
hCG

O   20   40
Weeks of pregnancy   Parturition

Mature ovum with corona radiata

Male pronucleus
Female pronucleus
Beginning of cell division of the ovum

Secretes → hCG
ACTH
hPL
Syncytiotrophoblast
Cytotrophoblast
Fetus
Secretes
GnRH
CRH
TRH
Somatostatin
Inhibin
Fetoplacental unit

(b) Physiological actions of progesterone

Thermogenic

Vagina—inhibits estrogen-induced cornification

Physiological actions of progesterone

Mammary glands—limit prepartum actions of prolactin on lactogenesis

CNS—inhibits GnRH secretion; alters sexual receptivity

Oviducts—stimulate growth and development for gamete transport

Uterus

Endometrium—stimulates growth and development for implantation

Cervix—increases consistency of mucus

Myometrium—anti-estrogenic (decreases estrogen receptors); hyperpolarizes muscle; decreases sensitivity to oxytocin

(c) Estriol biosynthesis

		Estrone Estradiol		
Maternal	Cholesterol		DHEA-S	Estriol
	Cholesterol		DHEA-S	Estriol
Placental	Pregnenolone	Estrone Estradiol ← DHEA	16-Alpha-OH-DHEA-S
	Progesterone			
	Progesterone			
Fetal		Estrone Estradiol	DHEA-S (Adrenal)	16-Alpha-OH-DHEA-S (liver)
	Cholesterol			

Fertilization and implantation

The ovum and sperm pronuclei fuse to form the **zygote**, which now has the normal diploid chromosomal number (Fig. 27a). The zygote divides mitotically as it travels along the uterine tube, and at about 3 days after fertilization enters the uterus, when it is now a **morula**. The cells of the morula continue to divide to form a hollow sphere, the **early blastocyst**, consisting of a single layer of **trophoblast** cells and the **embryoblast**, an inner core of cells which will form the embryo. The trophoblast, after implantation, will form the vascular interface with the maternal circulation. After around 2 days in the uterus, the blastocyst is accepted by the endometrial epithelium under the influence of estrogens, progesterone and other endometrial factors. This embedding or implantation process triggers the 'decidual response', involving an expansion of a space, the decidua, to accommodate the embryo as it grows. The invasive trophoblast proliferates into a protoplasmic cell mass called a **syncitiotrophoblast**, which will eventually form the uteroplacental circulation. By about 10 days, the embryo is completely embedded in the endometrium.

If the ovum is fertilized and becomes implanted, the corpus luteum does not regress, but continues to secrete progesterone, and within 10–12 days after ovulation the syncitiotrophoblast begins to secrete **human chorionic gonadotrophin** (hCG) into the intervillous space. Most pregnancy tests are based on the detection of hCG, which takes over the role of luteinizing hormone (LH) and stimulates the production of progesterone, 17-hydroxyprogesterone and estradiol by the corpus luteum. Plasma levels of hCG reach a peak between the ninth and fourteenth week of pregnancy, when luteal function begins to fade, and by 20 weeks, both luteal function and plasma hCG have declined.

The syncitiotrophoblast secretes another hormone, **human placental lactogen** (hPL), whose plasma levels in the maternal circulation (but not in that of the fetus) rise concomitantly with placental growth. Its function may be to inhibit maternal growth hormone production, and it has several metabolic effects, notably glucose-sparing and lipolytic, possibly through its anti-insulin effects. As a result, the placenta ensures a plentiful supply of glucose, free fatty acids and amino acids for the fetus.

The corpus luteum synthesizes **relaxin**, which relaxes the uterine muscle. The hormone is detected in the ovarian venous drainage, is present throughout pregnancy, rising in late gestation, but is rarely found in the plasma of non-pregnant women. Relaxin targets the pubic symphysis, that is the point of fusion of the pubic bones, and softens this by converting the connective tissues from a hard to a more fluid consistency. This will facilitate the widening of the pubis to allow the fetus to pass through. Relaxin achieves this effect by increasing the secretion of two enzymes, collagenase and plasminogen activator, both of which dissolve collagen. In late pregnancy, relaxin may be synthesized by the myometrium, the decidua (the mucous membrane which lines the pregnant uterus) and by the placenta.

The placenta, which takes over the production of the hormones of pregnancy from the corpus luteum, is part of what is termed the fetoplacental unit. The placenta attains its mature structure by the end of the first trimester of pregnancy. Its functional unit is the chorionic villus, consisting of a central core of loose connective tissue, packed with capillaries which communicate with the fetal circulation. Around the core are two layers of trophoblast, an inner layer of cytotrophoblast cells and an outer syncytium. The placenta is not only an endocrine organ, but also provides nutrients for the developing fetus and removes its waste products. The fetoplacental unit produces many of the hormones released by the hypothalamic–pituitary–gonadal axis.

Steroidogenesis

Progesterone concentrations rise progressively during pregnancy, and a major function of the hormone is thought to be its action, together with relaxin, to inhibit uterine motility, partly by decreasing its sensitivity to oxytocin (Fig. 27b). The placenta lacks 17-hydroxylase and therefore cannot produce androgens. This is done by the fetal adrenal glands, and the androgens thus formed are the precursors of the estrogens. The placenta converts maternal and fetal dehydroepiandrosterone sulphate (DHEA-S) to testosterone and androstenedione, which are aromatized to estrone and estradiol.

Another enzyme lacking in the placenta is 16-hydroxylase, so the placenta cannot directly form estriol and needs DHEA-S as substrate. Estriol formed by the placenta (Fig. 27c) passes into the maternal circulation, where it is conjugated in the liver to form the more soluble estriol glucuronides, which are excreted in the urine, and levels of estriol are used as an index of normal fetal development. If the fetus lacks a pituitary gland, no ACTH is produced and no DHEA-S, and therefore no estriol. The consequences of estriol deficiency are delayed labour and intrauterine death, unless caesarean section is carried out. Such mothers are resistant to oxytocin administration, suggesting a deficiency of oxytocin receptors, which are normally induced at term by estradiol. Another important role of estrogens is to stimulate the steady rise in maternal plasma **prolactin**. Prolactin, which is the postpartum lactogenic hormone, may serve in pregnancy to regulate storage and mobilization of fat, and to aid in maintaining metabolic homeostasis during pregnancy.

28 Female reproduction: IV Parturition and lactation

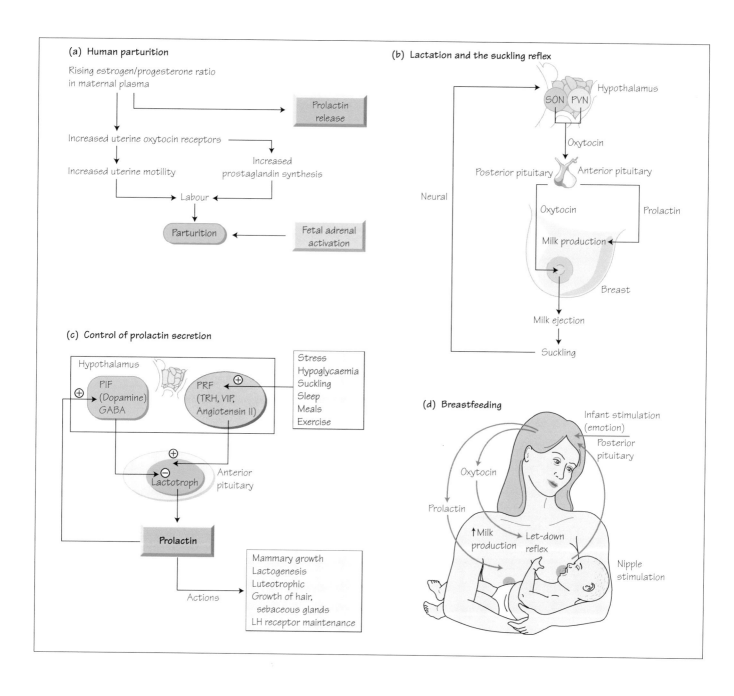

(a) Human parturition

Rising estrogen/progesterone ratio in maternal plasma
→ Prolactin release
→ Increased uterine oxytocin receptors → Increased prostaglandin synthesis
→ Increased uterine motility
→ Labour
→ Parturition ← Fetal adrenal activation

(b) Lactation and the suckling reflex

Hypothalamus — SON PVN
Oxytocin
Posterior pituitary — Anterior pituitary
Oxytocin — Prolactin
Milk production
Breast
Milk ejection
Neural
Suckling

(c) Control of prolactin secretion

Hypothalamus
PIF (Dopamine) GABA ⊕
PRF (TRH, VIP, Angiotensin II) ⊕
Stress
Hypoglycaemia
Suckling
Sleep
Meals
Exercise
⊕ Lactotroph ⊖
Anterior pituitary
Prolactin
Actions →
Mammary growth
Lactogenesis
Luteotrophic
Growth of hair, sebaceous glands
LH receptor maintenance

(d) Breastfeeding

Infant stimulation (emotion)
Posterior pituitary
Oxytocin
Prolactin
↑Milk production
Let-down reflex
Nipple stimulation

Parturition and lactation

The factors that stimulate parturition (birth) in humans are complex, and reflect a synchronized set of endocrine-related events (Fig. 28a). As estrogen levels rise during pregnancy, they stimulate an increase in uterine oxytocin receptors. The fetus grows rapidly near to the time of birth; its hypothalamus–pituitary system matures and activates the adrenal system, resulting in increased secretion of cortisol, and there is evidence that the fetus produces the oxytocin necessary for the onset of labour.

Cortisol is known to be important in the initiation of labour in some mammals, for example the sheep, but it is not known if fetal cortisol plays a similarly pivotal role in human parturition. The distension of the uterus caused by fetal growth may also contribute to increased oxytocin receptor synthesis. Oxytocin, through its receptors, may also stimulate prostaglandin (Pg) synthesis, particularly of PgF_2 and PgE_2. The prostaglandins are a group of oxygenated, unsaturated, long-chain fatty acids with profound effects on virtually all tissues, and PgE_2 and PgF_2 appear to act through the cAMP second messenger system to increase cytosolic Ca^{2+} and thus uterine contractility. These two have a therapeutic role in the induction of labour. During parturition, there is a profound fall in maternal plasma estrogen and progesterone concentrations, but it is not known what causes the rapid and sudden changes in the secretion of the female sex hormones during labour.

There is evidence that nitric acid donors ripen the human uterine cervix and the enzyme nitric oxide synthase is upregulated during spontaneous human cervical ripening. Inflammatory mediators may play an important role as well. The onset of labour is associated with a large influx of leukocytes, mainly T lymphocytes, neutrophils and macrophages, into the myometrium.

Lactation and the suckling reflex

Although maternal prolactin (PRL) plasma levels rise well before birth, their role in pregnancy is unknown. During pregnancy the breast enlarges, due to the combined effects of PRL, placental lactogen, cortisol, growth hormone, estrogens and progesterone on the growth of the mammary lobular–alveolar system, but lactogenesis is virtually absent. Estrogen and progesterone actually inhibit milk production through a direct inhibitory effect on PRL receptor synthesis.

After birth, however, the concentrations of these two sex hormones are relatively low, and PRL is allowed to play its key role in promoting lactogenesis. Lactogenesis and milk secretion begin very soon after birth. Milk is produced in the cells which line the alveoli, and is composed of lactose (produced from glucose), milk proteins, the most important of which are casein and whey, lipids, divalent cations, and also antibodies, through which the mother temporarily transfers certain forms of immunity to the baby. In humans, certain drugs are also carried in breast milk and this may be an important consideration for women on long-term medication such as antiepileptics or those using, for example, drugs of addiction.

There is evidence that PRL stimulates milk production through stimulation of the phospholipase A_2 second messenger system and increased prostaglandin synthesis, resulting in increased mRNA for casein. Cortisol and insulin are essential for this action of PRL. PRL has also been shown to activate the transport of K^+ and Na^+ through an action on the Na^+/Ka^+–ATPase pump, which in mammary tissue is confined mainly to the basolateral membranes of the mammary epithelial cells.

The suckling reflex. PRL secretion from the anterior pituitary lactotroph cell is controlled by a reflex, the neuroendocrine **suckling reflex** (Fig. 28b). The secretion of prolactin is normally under the inhibitory control of **dopamine** (called prolactin-inhibitory factor, or PIF) from the hypothalamus. The neurotransmitter gamma-aminobutyric acid (GABA) may mediate the release of PIF (Fig. 28c). When a mother begins nursing, or suckling the baby, the mechanical stimulation of the nipple sends afferent impulses through the anterolateral columns of the spinal cord, some of which converge, eventually, in the supraoptic (SON) and paraventricular (PVN) nuclei in the hypothalamus. Oxytocin is released from neurosecretory terminals in the posterior pituitary, and travels in the bloodstream to the mammary gland, where it contracts the mammary myoepithelial cells, resulting in an explosive discharge of milk. The same reflex somehow lessens or removes the inhibitory influence of dopamine, resulting in PRL release from the anterior pituitary.

The control of prolactin release by the brain is complex and not fully understood. A novel prolactin-releasing peptide has been described in the hypothalamus, but its role as a specific PRL-releasing factor is not established. Thyrotrophin-releasing hormone (TRH), vasoinhibitory peptide (VIP) and angiotensin II act in the hypothalamus to stimulate PRL secretion from the anterior pituitary. Milk production is maintained for as long as nursing is continued. In some poorer societies, a mother may lactate for up to 3 years, during which time she is relatively infertile. During nursing, gonadotrophin secretion from the pituitary is inhibited, and sex hormone production remains low. This results in a form of natural contraception. Non-lactating women will return to normal cyclic activity within about 4–5 weeks after birth, whereas in lactating women there will be no ovarian follicular development while plasma PRL levels remain elevated. After weaning, or the cessation of suckling, the secretion of estradiol and of LH increases, reflecting the resumption of normal ovarian function.

Prolactin has many other actions in both males and females, many of which are still poorly understood. It is released in stress, sleep, during eating and exercise, and is involved in hair growth. During the normal menstrual cycle it appears to maintain LH receptor production, and also to maintain LH receptors during pregnancy.

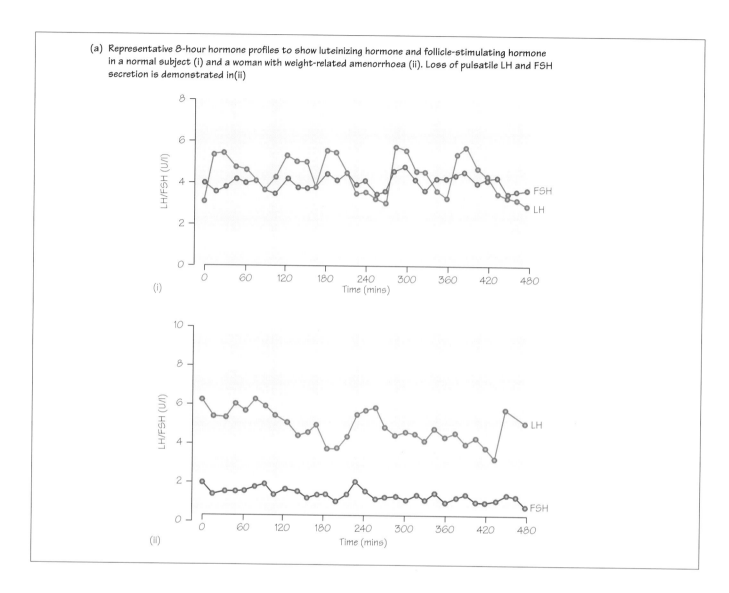

(a) Representative 8-hour hormone profiles to show luteinizing hormone and follicle-stimulating hormone in a normal subject (i) and a woman with weight-related amenorrhoea (ii). Loss of pulsatile LH and FSH secretion is demonstrated in(ii)

Clinical scenario

A 19-year-old history student, CV, presented to her university health centre requesting oral contraception. The GP noticed that she appeared very thin and enquired about her menstrual history. CV explained that her periods started when she was 15 and although she had regular cycles for about 1 year, during her time in the 6th form they had become very intermittent and had finally stopped altogether when she was 17. She was conscious of her appearance and liked being thin. She had started running for exercise during her schooldays and generally ran 10 miles four or five times a week and went to the gym several times weekly. On examination her body mass index was 16.5 kg/m². She had normal secondary sexual characteristics and there were no other abnormal physical findings. Biochemistry showed LH 1.2 U/L, FSH 0.9 U/L, estradiol 54 nmol/L and prolactin 235 mU/L. A diagnosis of hypothalamic amenorrhoea associated with low weight and excessive exercise was made. After discussion she agreed to try and gain weight and 1 year later her body mass index was 20.5 kg/m² and her periods had resumed.

Reproductive pathophysiology

Disorders of reproductive function in females present with menstrual irregularity (Table 29.1).

Primary amenorrhoea and delayed puberty should always be investigated as in the majority of cases a serious underlying cause will be found and must be treated (Table 29.2).

Secondary amenorrhoea. There are a number of causes of secondary amenorrhoea (Table 29.3), all of which rarely present

Table 29.1

Type	Characteristics
Primary amenorrhoea	Definition – absence of menses by the age of 16 years
	Rare – all cases should be thoroughly investigated
	Causes of secondary amenorrhoea may present as primary amenorrhoea
Secondary amenorrhoea	Definition – absence of menses for 6 months or more in a woman who has previously menstruated
	Common – important to exclude rare disorders of the hypothalamo–pituitary–ovarian axis
Oligomenorrhoea	Definition – irregular, infrequent menstrual cycles with no discernible cycle pattern
	Common – PCOS most frequent diagnosis

Table 29.2 Causes of primary amenorrhoea

Disorder	Example
Gonadal dysgenesis	Turner syndrome
	Other rare forms of gonadal dysgenesis
Genital tract dysgenesis	
Disorders of genital differentiation	True hermaphroditism
	Male and female pseudohermaphroditism
Ovarian insensitivity syndromes	
Gonadal irradiation or chemotherapy	
Hypothalamic–pituitary disease	Hypogonadotrophic hypogonadism
	Combined pituitary hormone deficiencies
	Radiotherapy/chemotherapy
	Hypothalamic–pituitary tumours
Delayed puberty	Constitutional delay
	Chronic illness
	Psychological disorders
Polycystic ovary syndrome	

Table 29.3 Causes of secondary amenorrhoea

Disorder	Example
Primary ovarian failure	Autoimmune ovarian failure
	Resistant ovary syndromes
	Radiotherapy/chemotherapy
	Postinfectious
	Postoperative
	Gonadal dysgenesis
Secondary ovarian failure	Hyperprolactinaemia
	Hypothalamic–pituitary tumours
	Empty sella syndrome
	Sheehan's syndrome
	Radiotherapy/chemotherapy
	Postoperative
Functional disorders	Weight loss-related amenorrhoea
	Exercise-related amenorrhoea
	Psychogenic
	Severe illness
	Idiopathic hypogonadotrophic hypogonadism
Polycystic ovary syndrome	
Genital tract disorders	
Ovarian tumours	Androgen secreting
	Estrogen secreting

as primary amenorrhoea. In all cases, careful history and examination is essential, combined with appropriate endocrine investigations to establish the cause. Patients with primary ovarian failure may have a history of other autoimmune disorders or of previous therapy for malignant disease. Patients with prolactinomas usually present with associated features of prolactin excess, such as galactorrhoea.

Hypothalamic amenorrhoea. The term 'functional disorders' is used to describe a group of conditions in which there are no structural or endocrine synthetic abnormalities in the pituitary–ovarian axis. Hypothalamic amenorrhoea is usually associated with weight-reducing diets, often with excess exercise in an attempt to remain slim, and is seen in athletes, in subjects with anorexia nervosa and in other forms of stress, either physical or psychological in origin. It is the commonest cause of secondary amenorrhoea seen in endocrine clinics.

Although a reduction in weight to 10% below ideal body weight is usually associated with amenorrhoea, there is wide variation between women. Changes in body composition, particularly reduced fat mass, are crucial to the characteristic hypothalamic changes of impaired GnRH secretion, loss of gonadotrophin pulsatility and subsequent hypogonadotrophic hypogonadism (Fig. 29a).

The treatment of weight- and exercise-related amenorrhoea is specifically weight gain and reduction in exercise. These measures restore normal ovulatory cycles and reproductive potential but may require lengthy treatment with a multidisciplinary team of endocrinologists, dieticians and psychologists. Untreated, hypothalamic amenorrhoea is associated with reduced bone mineral density and ultimately osteoporosis. Women with long-term hypoestrogenaemia should have their bone density recorded and, if there is significant osteopaenia or osteoporosis, combined estrogen/progesterone replacement therapy should be considered.

Polycystic ovary syndrome. Patients with polycystic ovary syndrome (PCOS) or non-classical congenital adrenal hyperplasia usually present with oligomenorrhoea and other signs of androgen excess (Chapter 26). Treatment is aimed at the symptoms of hyperandrogenaemia and restoring ovulatory menstrual cycles where fertility is the goal. Women with PCOS may also demonstrate other features of hyperinsulinaemia, including obesity and low HDL-cholesterol levels. In the long term, the risks of Type 2 diabetes and cardiovascular disease are increased and weight reduction and exercise play an important role in the clinical management of these patients.

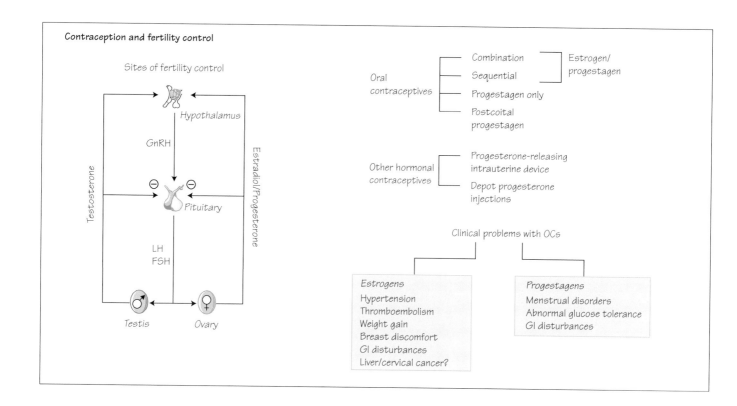

Contraception and fertility control

Sites of fertility control

Hypothalamus

GnRH

Testosterone

Estradiol/Progesterone

Pituitary

LH
FSH

Testis   Ovary

Oral contraceptives
- Combination — Estrogen/progestagen
- Sequential — Estrogen/progestagen
- Progestagen only
- Postcoital progestagen

Other hormonal contraceptives
- Progesterone-releasing intrauterine device
- Depot progesterone injections

Clinical problems with OCs

Estrogens
Hypertension
Thromboembolism
Weight gain
Breast discomfort
GI disturbances
Liver/cervical cancer?

Progestagens
Menstrual disorders
Abnormal glucose tolerance
GI disturbances

Clinical background

There are many oral contraceptive preparations on the market and a choice should be made to prescribe the one with the lowest estrogen and progesterone concentrations that give good cycle control. Combined oral contraceptives (COCs) can also be used to treat a number of gynaecological conditions involving irregular cycles, menorrhagia or dysmenorrhoea. In addition to progesterone only pills (POPs), intrauterine devices which release progesterone locally to the endometrium are available (Mirena Intrauterine Systems, Schering Health) and are used both for contraception and for the treatment of endometriosis and other painful disorders of menstruation.

COCs are contraindicated in women who are pregnant, or who have a history of various forms of cardiovascular disease, cerebrovascular problems, certain liver disorders and undiagnosed gynaecological problems. COCs influence blood coagulation and there is a small increased risk of deep vein thrombosis, pulmonary embolism, stroke and myocardial infarction. This is slightly higher in women taking COCs containing third-generation progestagens (desogestrel, gestodene), particularly when there are other risk factors such as obesity, smoking and older age (>35 years). COCs should not be prescribed to women with known clotting abnormalities or a history of hemiplegic migraine. Side-effects should be monitored including regular blood pressure readings.

Oral contraceptives

Oral contraception is fertility control using orally active synthetic sex hormone derivatives (Fig. 30a).

Combined oral contraceptives (COCs) represent the most widely used form of estrogens and progestagens, and constitute the most reliable and effective method for preventing pregnancy in countries where they are widely available. COCs act by preventing ovulation through negative-feedback inhibition of gonadotrophin release. Women taking COCs do not show the early follicular rise of follicle-stimulating hormone (FSH), nor the midcycle rises in FSH and luteinizing hormone (LH). The COC is taken daily for 21 days and withheld for seven, to induce withdrawal bleeding. The COC may also act directly on the uterus and cervix. Cervical mucus becomes more viscous, presumably inhibiting penetration by sperm, and the endometrium does not develop into a suitable matrix for implantation.

Sequential COCs are prescribed so that the user takes estrogen alone daily for 14–16 days, then estrogen and progestagen together for 5–6 days, then 7 days without any pills; this aims to mimic the natural cycle.

Advantages of COC use. COCs provide reliable, reversible contraception and have a number of other advantages such as reduced dysmenorrhoea and menorrhagia, less benign breast disease and a reduced risk of ovarian and endometrial cancer.

Disdvantages of COC use. There is a small increase in the rate of venous thromboembolism in all women taking COCs and a history of thromboembolic disease or other risk factors for thromboembolism, such as obesity, immobility or a family history, are contraindications to this form of contraception. Likewise, there is an increased risk of arterial vascular disease and the COC should be avoided for older women, particularly smokers with obesity and/or hypertension. Other relative contraindications include migraine and a number of rare liver disorders. COCs should not be given to women with a history of breast or genital tract cancer.

Progestagen only pills (POPs; mini-pills) were introduced to eliminate the adverse effects reported with estrogen use. The progestagen does inhibit FSH and LH release but a major component of action is due to the thickening of cervical mucus, and endometrial atrophy. The method is not as reliable as COCs, the success rate being 97–98%, as opposed to 99% for combination OC use. Adverse effects reported with progestagen only OCs are: amenorrhoea; changes in plasma high-density lipoprotein (HDL) and low-density lipoprotein (LDL) – HDL decrease and LDL increase in concentration in plasma; breakthrough bleeding and 'spotting'; and abnormal responses to glucose tolerance tests.

Emergency contraception is prescribed as levonorgestrel and is effective if the first dose is taken within 72 hours of unprotected intercourse. The treatment creates an endometrial environment hostile to the blastocyst and is followed by a withdrawal bleed that may be heavy.

Other uses of estrogens

Hormone replacement therapy (HRT) describes the use of sex hormones to replace the lack of endogenous hormones resulting from the cessation of cyclicity of ovarian function at the menopause or in women who have developed hypogonadism for other reasons. HRT is administered in the form of sequential daily doses of estrogen, coupled with progesterone in women with an intact uterus to prevent the risk of endometrial hyperplasia and malignancy. There are numerous HRT preparations in the form of tablets, transdermal patches and creams. The benefit versus risk of HRT should be calculated in all symptomatic menopausal women and it should not be prescribed for longer than 5–10 years, following which the risks from breast cancer and cardiovascular disease increase. In the absence of good data to the contrary, hypogonadal women should be treated up until the expected age of the menopause.

31 Male reproduction: I The testis

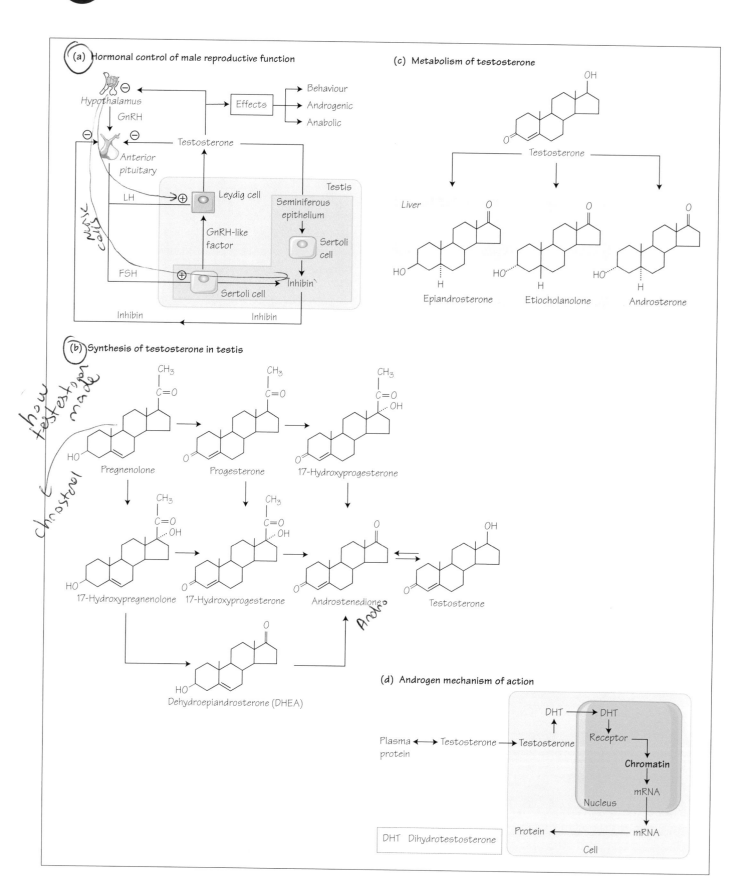

(a) Hormonal control of male reproductive function

(c) Metabolism of testosterone

(b) Synthesis of testosterone in testis

(d) Androgen mechanism of action

DHT Dihydrotestosterone

Clinical background

Normal fertility in the male is produced by a complex interaction between genetic, autocrine, paracrine and endocrine function. The endocrine control of reproductive function in the male depends upon an intact hypothalamo–pituitary–testicular axis. The testis has a dual role – the production of spermatozoa and the synthesis and secretion of testosterone needed for the development and maintenance of secondary sexual characteristics and essential for maintaining spermatogenesis. These functions in turn depend upon the pituitary gonadotrophin hormones: luteinizing hormone (LH; required to stimulate testicular Leydig cells to produce testosterone); and follicle stimulating hormone (FSH; required for the development of the immature testis and a possible role in adult spermatogenesis). Gonadotrophin production occurs in response to stimulation by hypothalamic GnRH. Testosterone exerts a negative feedback on the secretion of LH and FSH and the hormone inhibin-β, also synthesized by the testis, has a specific regulatory role for FSH. Thus in primary seminiferous tubular failure, low testosterone concentrations are associated with elevated gonadotrophins whereas in the presence of hypothalamic pituitary disease the gonadotrophin concentrations are low (secondary testicular failure).

Spermatogenesis is dependent upon testosterone availability. In primary seminiferous tubular failure androgen deficiency has a number of causes including: genetic defects in the Y chromosome and gonadotrophin receptor genes, previous testicular inflammation such as mumps orchitis and chemotherapy or radiotherapy for malignant disease. Patients exhibit signs of androgen deficiency and the azoospermia is associated with elevated gonadotrophin levels (hypergonadotrophic hypogonadism). Treatment requires androgen replacement therapy with assessment and management in a specialist fertility treatment centre.

The testis

The testis is the male gonad, and its primary functions are the production of spermatozoa and testosterone. The spermatozoa are produced in the seminiferous tubules and testosterone is synthesized in the Leydig cell. In the human male, the two testes are in the scrotum, each about 5 cm in length and about 2–3 cm in diameter. The testis is encapsulated within a connective tissue sheath called the tunica albuginea, and consists chiefly of a packed mass of convoluted seminiferous tubules. In each testis, these converge into the rete testis, which opens to feed ductules to the epididymis. The epididymis has a head and a tail, the latter feeding into the vas deferens.

The seminiferous tubules consist of an outer sheath of connective and smooth muscle, surrounding an inner lining containing the Sertoli cells. Embedded within and between the Sertoli cells are the germ cells which produce the spermatozoa. These are released into the lumen of the tubule and are stored in the tail of the epididymis. The Leydig cells, also called the intestitial cells, lie between the seminiferous tubules and secrete testosterone.

Control of testis function (Fig. 31a). The hypothalamus sends episodic pulses (approximately once every 90 minutes) of gonadotrophin releasing hormone (GnRH) to the anterior pituitary gonadotroph cells, which secrete follicle-stimulating hormone (FSH) and luteinizing hormone (LH) (Chapter 5). LH targets the Leydig cell, where it stimulates testosterone production through the cAMP second messenger system. FSH targets the Sertoli cell, where, together with testosterone, it stimulates cAMP and subsequent spermatogenesis. There is evidence that FSH, perhaps together with **prolactin**, increases the number of LH receptors on Leydig cells. Another hormone, **inhibin**, is produced by the testis, probably by the Sertoli cell. Inhibin, a polypeptide, inhibits FSH release from the pituitary gland by a negative feedback effect.

Testosterone biosynthesis in the Leydig cell is from cholesterol, which is converted to pregnenolone (Fig. 31b). In humans, most of the pregnenolone is 17-hydroxylated and then undergoes side-chain cleavage to yield the 17-ketosteroids, which are converted to testosterone. Once in the blood, approximately 95% of the testosterone is bound to plasma proteins, mainly to sex hormone-binding globulin (SHBG) and to albumin. Testosterone is metabolized to inactive metabolites chiefly in the liver. These are androsterone and etiocholanolone (Fig. 31c), which are excreted as soluble glucuronides and sulphates.

Testosterone mechanism of action. Testosterone acts not only as a hormone in its own right, but also as a **prohormone**. In the target cell, testosterone may be reduced to its 5-α-reduced metabolite 5-α-dihydrotestosterone (DHT; Fig. 31d), and also aromatized to estradiol. In a highly androgen-dependent tissue such as the prostate, testosterone diffuses into the cell, where it is converted to 5-α-dihydrotestosterone. This is the active androgen in the prostate gland. DHT binds to an intranuclear androgen receptor which stimulates transcription. The androgen receptor is also able to bind testosterone, and, to a lesser extent, progesterone. In this regard, it is worth mentioning that the androgen receptor exhibits a high structural homology with the receptor for progesterone, although they are distinct receptor types within the larger subfamily of steroid receptors (see Chapter 4). The androgen receptor possesses a hormone-binding domain and a DNA-binding region, consisting of two zinc fingers (see Chapter 4).

Antiandrogens have been synthesized which compete with DHT for its receptor site. These antiandrogens are based on the structure of progesterone, and examples include **cyproterone**, **cyproterone acetate** (CA) and **flutamide**. In human males, CA causes atrophy of the prostate and seminal vesicles, and a loss of libido. CA will inhibit the progress of acne in teenagers. In women, CA has been used to treat virilization and hirsutism in patients with polycystic ovary syndrome (Chapter 29). The 5α-reductase inhibitor **finasteride** is also effective.

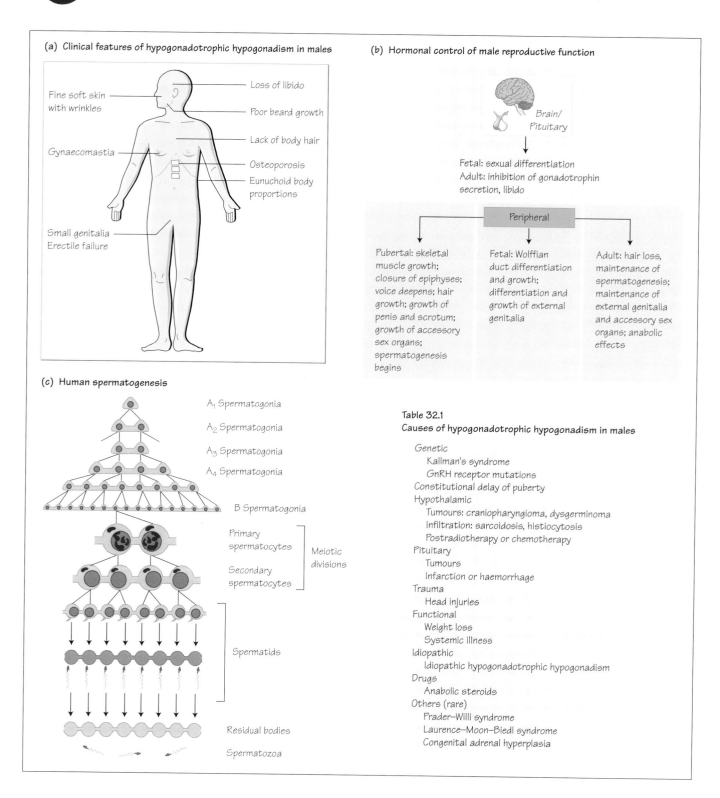

(a) Clinical features of hypogonadotrophic hypogonadism in males

Fine soft skin with wrinkles

Gynaecomastia

Small genitalia
Erectile failure

Loss of libido

Poor beard growth

Lack of body hair

Osteoporosis

Eunuchoid body proportions

(b) Hormonal control of male reproductive function

Brain/ Pituitary

Fetal: sexual differentiation
Adult: inhibition of gonadotrophin secretion, libido

Peripheral

Pubertal: skeletal muscle growth; closure of epiphyses; voice deepens; hair growth; growth of penis and scrotum; growth of accessory sex organs; spermatogenesis begins

Fetal: Wolffian duct differentiation and growth; differentiation and growth of external genitalia

Adult: hair loss, maintenance of spermatogenesis; maintenance of external genitalia and accessory sex organs; anabolic effects

(c) Human spermatogenesis

A_1 Spermatogonia
A_2 Spermatogonia
A_3 Spermatogonia
A_4 Spermatogonia

B Spermatogonia

Primary spermatocytes

Secondary spermatocytes

Meiotic divisions

Spermatids

Residual bodies

Spermatozoa

Table 32.1
Causes of hypogonadotrophic hypogonadism in males

Genetic
    Kallman's syndrome
    GnRH receptor mutations
Constitutional delay of puberty
Hypothalamic
    Tumours: craniopharyngioma, dysgerminoma
    Infiltration: sarcoidosis, histiocytosis
    Postradiotherapy or chemotherapy
Pituitary
    Tumours
    Infarction or haemorrhage
Trauma
    Head injuries
Functional
    Weight loss
    Systemic illness
Idiopathic
    Idiopathic hypogonadotrophic hypogonadism
Drugs
    Anabolic steroids
Others (rare)
    Prader–Willi syndrome
    Laurence–Moon–Biedl syndrome
    Congenital adrenal hyperplasia

Clinical scenario

Effects of the failure of androgen action may be best seen in patients with hypogonadotrophic hypogonadism (Fig. 32a). This is caused by a failure of hypothalamic GnRH secretion or by pituitary disease resulting in impaired gonadotrophin release and hence low androgen concentrations (Table 32.1). The clinical features of hypogonadotrophic hypogonadism depend on the timing of its onset, such that males developing the condition after puberty present with features of secondary testicular failure (poor libido, loss of secondary sexual characteristics and subfertility). Prior to puberty, boys present with delayed or failed puberty or, less commonly, the condition presents in the neonatal period with cryptorchidism and micropenis Idiopathic hypogonadotrophic hypogonadism describes those patients in whom there are no anatomical abnormalities of the hypothalamus and pituitary and no associated endocrine disorders.

AB presented to the endocrine clinic at the age of 16 years. He had symptoms of delayed puberty, with absence of secondary sexual characteristics, but had always been as tall as his friends at school. On questioning he thought his sense of smell was poor and his parents confirmed this observation. On examination his height was on the 75th centile for age but pubertal assessment revealed no evidence of sexual maturation. Formal testing of the first cranial nerve showed anosmia. Hypogonadotrophic hypogonadism was confirmed biochemically – LH 0.4 U/L, FSH 0.6 U/L, testosterone 5.3 nmol/L, prolactin 145 mU/L, TFTs and cortisol were normal. An MRI scan confirmed a normal pituitary gland and detailed MRI scans of the hypothalamus revealed abnormalities consistent with Kallman's syndrome. He was subsequently treated with gonadotrophins to induce pubertal development. Kallman's syndrome is caused by the failure of migration of GnRH neurones from the olfactory bulb to the arcuate nucleus of the hypothalamus in early fetal life. Both X-linked and autosomal forms of the disorder have been described and may be associated with other midline defects and synkinesia.

Actions of testosterone

The actions of testosterone (Fig. 32b) are to establish and maintain the function of the male and to maintain libido in the female. The actions of testosterone can be broadly classified as **androgenic** and **anabolic**.

Brain and spinal cord. In birds and mammals, testosterone sexually differentiates the fetal brain. The fetal brain contains androgen and estrogen receptors, which mediate these actions of testosterone. In fetal rats, testosterone may act to protect neurones from cell death.

In adult male rats, the medial preoptic nuclei in the brain are larger than in females, but this difference is eliminated if the males are castrated during the critical period of brain sexual differentiation. Conversely, if neonatal female rats are injected with testosterone, they develop a medial preoptic region similar in size to that of the male. Castration of an adult rat results in the shrinkage of cell bodies and axons of motor neurones involved in male copulation, and these are restored in size after androgen replacement. Although no evidence is available about these actions of testosterone in humans, there is evidence that testosterone causes changes in the fetal brain during sexual differentiation of the brain at about 6 weeks.

Behaviour. The precise nature of the influence of testosterone on behaviour is unknown, due in part to the limitations of methods of study. In humans, there is no apparent relationship between plasma levels of testosterone and sexual or aggressive behaviour. It seems that behaviour has a powerful influence on testosterone production, since stress drives it down, as does depression and threatening behaviour from others. In captive primate colonies, subordinate males have raised prolactin and very much reduced plasma levels of testosterone.

Peripheral actions of testosterone

A fundamental role of testosterone, together with follicle-stimulating hormone (FSH), is the maintenance of spermatogenesis. It is currently believed that FSH stimulates Sertoli cells to produce cAMP, which stimulates synthesis of a specific protein, androgen-binding protein (ABP), which is secreted into the lumen of the seminiferous tubules. The Sertoli cells also produce the nutrient requirements of the growing and differentiating spermatozoa. Luteinizing hormone (LH) stimulates the Leydig cells to produce testosterone, which binds to ABP, and the complex brings testosterone into close proximity with the developing spermatocytes. ABP may also function to build up local concentrations of testosterone and transport the hormone to the epididymis. The Leydig cell also synthesizes estrogens which bind to ABP, and which are essential for normal spermatogenesis. Growth hormone is essential for early division of the spermatogonia.

Spermatogenesis (Fig. 32c). About 120 million sperm are produced each day by the young adult human testis. Most are stored in the vas deferens and the ampulla of the vas deferens, where they can remain and retain their fertility for at least 1 month. While stored, they are inactive due to several inhibitory factors, and are activated once in the uterus. In the female reproductive tract, sperm remain alive for 1 or 2 days at most. Sperm remain alive in neutral or mildly alkaline environments, but are rapidly killed in strong acid media. The metabolic activity of sperm increases markedly with increasing temperature, but this also shortens their life considerably.

Accessory sex organs. Testosterone maintains the functions and structural integrity of the **seminal vesicles** and the **prostate gland**. The seminal vesicles are essentially secretory, producing many substances, including large quantities of prostaglandins, fructose and fibrinogen. During ejaculation, the seminal vesicles contract, ejecting their fluid into that carrying the spermatozoa. Fructose is an important nutrient for the sperm, and prostaglandins aid in the movement of sperm by contracting the uterus and uterine tubes, as well as by reacting with cervical mucus to make it receptive to sperm. During orgasm and emission, the prostate gland secretes a thin, alkaline fluid containing a profibrinolysin, a clotting enzyme, calcium, citrate ions and acidic phosphate. The functions of prostatic fluid are unknown, but they may serve to create a less acidic environment for the sperm and increase their motility.

Anabolic actions of testosterone. Testosterone increases basal metabolic rate through an increase in enzyme and other protein synthesis. Testosterone produces a 10–15% increase in red blood cell production during puberty, and men have about 700 000 more red blood cells per millilitre than women. Testosterone increases muscle mass, despite an apparent absence of androgen receptors in skeletal muscle. The effect may be due to an inhibition of the normal catabolic effects of glucocorticoids in muscle.

(a) Treatment of prostate cancer

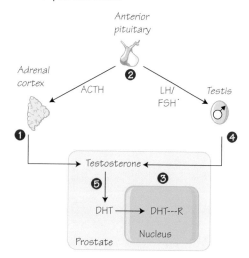

DES	Diethylstilboestrol
DHT	Dihydrotestosterone

❶ Ketoconazole
❷ DES or GnRH
❸ Flutamide
❹ Surgery (castrate)
❺ 5α-reductase inhibition

Table 33.1 Clinical aspects of male infertility

(adapted from Baker HWG. Management of male infertility. Ballieres Clinical Endocrinology and Metabolism 2000; 14(3): 409–422)

Condition	Clinical features	Investigations	Treatment options
Primary seminiferous tubule failure (genetic, inflammatory, chemotherapy/ radiotherapy in childhood)	History of orchitis or previous treatment for malignancy. Virilization and testicular size normal or reduced. May have undescended testes. features of genetic syndromes	Testosterone low. Gonadotropins high or normal. Persistent azoospermia	Androgen replacement therapy. Infertility untreatable – consider donor insemination or adoption
Reversible effects of toxins, drugs (e.g. salazopyrin), febrile illnesses, heat and chemicals	History of exposure	Endocrinology usually normal. Semen analysis variable and improves	Avoid exposure or treat illness. Monitor progress
Gonadotrophin deficiency or suppression (secondary testicular failure)	Reduced libido and virilization. Other features of hypothalamo-pituitary disease including Kallman's syndrome. Anabolic steroid abuse	Testosterone and gonadotrophins low. Check for hyperprolactinaemia and other features of pituitary tumour. Ferritin elevated in haemochromatosis. Oligo- or azoospermia	Treat pituitary disease. May require exogenous gonadotrophin therapy. Stop steroid abuse
Sperm autoimmunity	Other autoimmune disorders or family history of autoimmunity. Examination normal	Semen analysis variable. Postcoital test reveals poor semen penetration of cervical mucus. IgG and IgA antibodies	Intracytoplasmic sperm injection (ICSI). Glucocorticoids
Genital tract obstruction	History of sexually transmitted disease, vasectomy, other surgery, bronchiectasis or cystic fibrosis. Normal virilization	Gonadotrophins and testosterone normal. Azoospermia. Ultrasound may reveal genital tract abnormalities	Microsurgery or ICSI
Coital dysfunction	History of impotence or ejaculatory disorder. Low libido. Check other medication (e.g. beta bockers)	Exclude other causes of testosterone deficiency and neuro-vascular disease (diabetes)	Change medication. Counselling or other psychological management

Clinical background

Male infertility has a large number of causes, both endocrine and non-endocrine in origin and few are specifically treatable. In the majority of cases an exact diagnosis is not reached despite investigation and the condition may result from previous testicular damage, varicocoele or non-specific inflammation. All patients should be assessed with their partner in a specialist fertility unit and in the undiagnosed group the use of intracytoplasmic sperm injection may offer the best chance of fertility. The clinical features of male infertility are shown in Table 33.1.

Male reproductive pathophysiology

Hypogonadism is the failure of the testes to function, that is to produce testosterone and spermatozoa, and can be due to genetic defects (see Chapter 23). **Primary hypogonadism** refers to abnormalities within the gonad, for example Leydig cell agenesis (non-development), or failure of Leydig cells in adult life. Leydig cell failure can occur after mumps. **Secondary hypogonadism** refers to gonadotrophin deficiency or failure to secrete gonadotrophin-releasing hormone (GnRH), and is also called **hypogonadotrophic hypogonadism**.

Hypergonadism means the excess activity of the gonad, which can be **virilizing** due to androgen-secreting Leydig cell tumours, or **feminizing** due to estrogen-producing Leydig cell tumours. This is **primary hypergonadism**, whereas that produced through excess GnRH and/or gonadotrophin production is **secondary hypergonadism**.

Androgen resistance is caused by mutations of the androgen receptor, which no longer binds androgen with sufficient affinity for a normal androgenic response to be maintained, or by the complete absence of the androgen receptor.

Gynaecomastia is breast enlargement in males. It usually occurs through abnormal endogenous or exogenous estrogens. Gynaecomastia accompanied by galactorrhoea (milk production) may be indicative of a prolactin-secreting tumour. Gynaecomastia sometimes occurs in ageing men, which may be because of an increasing estrogen/ androgen ratio in the blood. The condition has also been reported after the smoking of cannabis, which is known to decrease testosterone synthesis and to drive down libido.

Impotence (erectile dysfunction) is the failure to achieve erection of the penis, and has numerous vascular and neurological causes, although few of endocrine origin. Erection is caused by nerve impulses passing through parasympathetic efferents, the nervi erigentes, to the penis. The result is vasodilatation of penile arteries, which allows the build-up of arterial blood in the corpus cavernosum and the corpus spongiosum.

The treatment of impotence was revolutionized by the introduction of sildenafil (Viagra). The drug dilates penile blood vessels by blocking the enzyme phosphodiesterase-5, which normally metabolizes the second messenger cyclic GMP, which in turn is permitted to prolong vascular smooth muscle relaxation in the penis, which is thus engorged with blood.

Prostatic pathophysiology

Benign prostatic hyperplasia (BPH) is the growth of the medial lobe of the human prostate, most often in late middle-aged men, until it presses on and begins to occlude the urethra. It is termed 'benign' because it does not invade other tissues and destroy them, or metastasize to distant sites in the body. BPH is androgen-dependent, being strongly stimulated by dihydrotestosterone (DHT), the active androgenic metabolite of testosterone in the prostate gland. The most effective treatment has been the surgical removal of all or part of the gland. The operation can be performed through the bladder (transvesical prostatectomy) or through the urethra (transurethral resection), when prostate tissue is burned away using a heated element. Recently, inhibitors of the enzyme 5α-reductase, which converts testosterone to DHT, have been introduced to treat BPH.

Prostate cancer. Carcinoma of the prostate is virtually always androgen-dependent. Various approaches to treatment are shown in Fig. 33a. The aim is to remove the tumour and all sources of androgen production. Medical treatment may involve the administration of stable analogues of GnRH, such as **buserelin**. These, if continuously present in the bloodstream, down regulate anterior pituitary production of gonadotrophins by rendering the gonadotrophs insensitive to GnRH from the hypothalamus. The result is a chemical castration, which can be reversed by stopping treatment. Another approach is the administration of androgen receptor blockers such as **flutamide**, **finasteride** or **cyproterone acetate**.

When using GnRH analogues, it is advisable when starting treatment to administer the drug together with an antiandrogen. This is because the initial effect of the GnRH analogue is to stimulate a transient increase in testosterone production, which may in turn cause stimulation of tumour activity. Radiotherapy may be necessary as an adjunctive therapy or for the relief of pain due to metastatic spread.

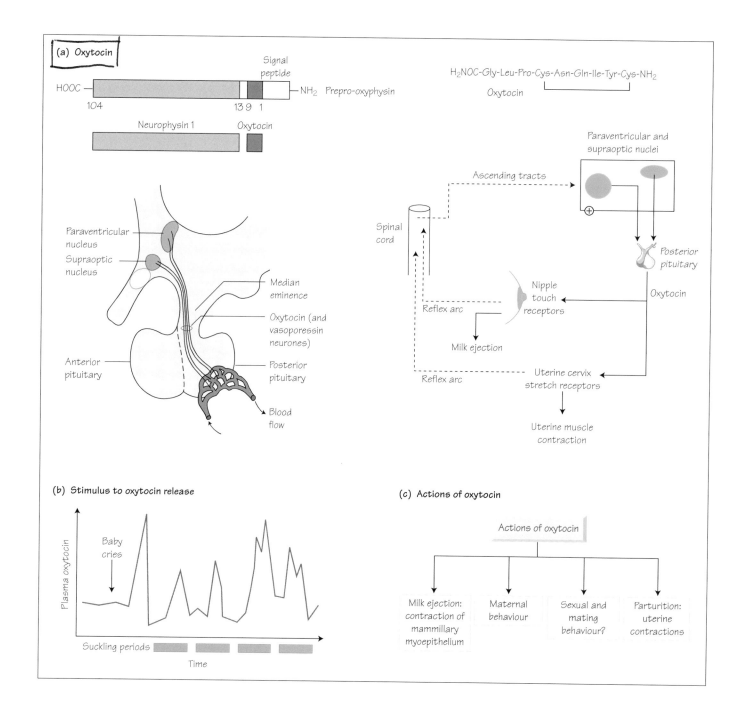

(a) Oxytocin

Signal peptide

HOOC — [Prepro-oxyphysin] — NH₂   Prepro-oxyphysin

104   13 9 1

Neurophysin 1   Oxytocin

$H_2NOC-Gly-Leu-Pro-Cys-Asn-Gln-Ile-Tyr-Cys-NH_2$

Oxytocin

Paraventricular nucleus
Supraoptic nucleus
Median eminence
Oxytocin (and vasoporessin neurones)
Anterior pituitary
Posterior pituitary
Blood flow

Paraventricular and supraoptic nuclei
Ascending tracts
Spinal cord
Posterior pituitary
Oxytocin
Nipple touch receptors
Reflex arc
Milk ejection
Reflex arc
Uterine cervix stretch receptors
Uterine muscle contraction

(b) Stimulus to oxytocin release

Plasma oxytocin
Baby cries
Suckling periods
Time

(c) Actions of oxytocin

Actions of oxytocin

Milk ejection: contraction of mammillary myoepithelium | Maternal behaviour | Sexual and mating behaviour? | Parturition: uterine contractions

Biosynthesis

Oxytocin is synthesized in the cell bodies of the magnocellular neurones of the paraventricular and supraoptic nuclei of the hypothalamus (Fig. 34a). Other neurones in the same nuclei produce vasopressin (see Chapter 35). The axons of these neurones pass through the median eminence and terminate in close contact with fenestrated capillaries in the posterior pituitary gland. Both oxytocin and vasopressin are synthesized in the rough endoplasmic reticulum of the cell body, together with proteins called **neurophysins**. Oxytocin and its neurophysin protein (called neurophysin I) are packaged together in the Golgi apparatus in the same vesicle or secretory granule. The vesicle also contains the enzymes which cleave oxytocin from the neurophysin as the granules migrate along the axon towards the nerve terminal. Neurophysin I is occasionally referred to as the oxytocin transport protein. There is evidence that if the neurophysins fail to be synthesized, then oxytocin and vasopressin do not reach the posterior pituitary. Chemically, oxytocin is a nonapeptide with a disulphide bridge between its two cysteine residues (Fig. 34a).

Oxytocin neurones send axons not only to the posterior pituitary, but also to higher centres in the brain, where the hormone may serve as a neurotransmitter mediating certain forms of behaviour (see below).

Secretion

Excitatory cholinergic and inhibitory neurones make synaptic contact with the neurosecretory oxytocin neurones in the paraventricular and supraoptic nuclei. Oxytocin is secreted from the nerve terminal by exocytosis, as a result of increased intracellular Ca^{2+}, due to depolarization of the axon membrane, which opens calcium channels. Oxytocin applied to the oxytocin neurones in the hypothalamus stimulates oxytocin release from the nerve terminals.

Actions

Oxytocin binds to its receptor on target cells, for example the mammary myoepithelium, uterine smooth muscle and brain and activates the phospholipase/inositol triphosphate (PLC/IP3) system, which increases intracellular calcium and the effect of the hormone is expressed.

Parturition. Oxytocin induces contraction of the smooth muscle of the uterine myometrium, during the last 2–3 weeks of pregnancy (Fig. 34a and c). This may be due to a sharp increase in the numbers of oxytocin receptors, whose synthesis is stimulated by the high circulating concentrations of estrogens present in the third trimester of pregnancy. The trigger for oxytocin receptor synthesis may be the increasing ratio of estrogen to progesterone, as concentrations of the latter hormone diminish during labour. Oxytocin is released from the posterior pituitary during the course of labour and parturition, possibly as a result of the dilation of the cervix, which sends afferent fibres to the central nervous system. It is not yet known whether the release of oxytocin is the *cause* of the onset of labour in humans.

Milk ejection. Suckling stimulates sensory nerve endings in the nipple and areolus of the breast, and the impulses are conducted along afferent fibres to the spinal cord (Fig. 34a), where they ascend via the lateral, dorsal and ventral spinothalamic tracts to the midbrain, from where excitatory fibres project directly to the oxytocin neurones in the hypothalamus and oxytocin is released from the pituitary gland. Oxytocin binds to receptors on the myoepithelial cells of the mammary tissue, causing contraction of their muscle-like fibres, and this increases intramammary pressure. Milk ejection from the breasts can occur even before the suckling reflex is initiated. The sound of a human baby crying may be sufficient to cause milk 'let down' (Fig. 34b).

Maternal behaviour can be elicited by oxytocin (Fig. 34c). If virgin rats are administered oxytocin directly into the cerebrospinal fluid, they exhibit maternal behaviour to foster pups. If the rats are ovariectomized, oxytocin no longer has the effect, which can be restored if the ovariectomized rats are first given injections of estrogen. Infusion of oxytocin into the ventricles of the brain of virgin rats or non-pregnant sheep rapidly induces maternal behaviour. Administration into the brain of oxytocin antibodies or of oxytocin antagonists prevents the maternal rat from accepting her pups. These experiments suggest that maternal behaviour results, at least in part, from exposure of the brain to high concentrations of estrogens, priming it for the action of oxytocin, which stimulates maternal behaviour, either as a neurotransmitter, or as a hormone or both. This is not to say that oxytocin is absolutely required for maternal behaviour. Rats in which the oxytocin gene was disrupted were still able to exhibit maternal behaviour, although suckling was severely impaired.

Other possible roles for oxytocin. Oxytocin is released from the human posterior pituitary during coitus and orgasm, but the significance of this, if any, remains unknown. Oxytocin may be involved in the facilitation of sperm transport. Oxytocin may also be involved in the mediation of, for example, anxiety and pair bonding in primates.

Oxytocin release is inhibited by, for example, acute stress, through the mediation of adrenal catecholamines, which bind to oxytocin neurones and inhibit oxytocin release.

35 Vasopressin = ADH

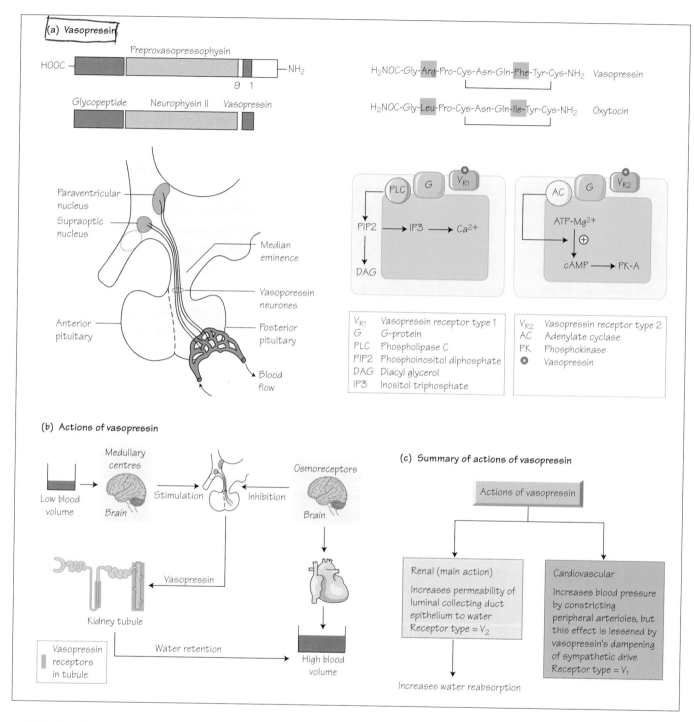

(a) Vasopressin

Preprovasopressophysin

HOOC — ... — NH₂

9 1

Glycopeptide   Neurophysin II   Vasopressin

H₂NOC-Gly-Arg-Pro-Cys-Asn-Gln-Phe-Tyr-Cys-NH₂   Vasopressin

H₂NOC-Gly-Leu-Pro-Cys-Asn-Gln-Ile-Tyr-Cys-NH₂   Oxytocin

Paraventricular nucleus
Supraoptic nucleus
Median eminence
Vasoporessin neurones
Anterior pituitary
Posterior pituitary
Blood flow

PLC G V_R1
PIP2 → IP3 → Ca²⁺
DAG

AC G V_R2
ATP-Mg²⁺
cAMP → PK-A

V_R1	Vasopressin receptor type 1
G	G-protein
PLC	Phospholipase C
PIP2	Phosphoinositol diphosphate
DAG	Diacyl glycerol
IP3	Inositol triphosphate

V_R2	Vasopressin receptor type 2
AC	Adenylate cyclase
PK	Phosphokinase
◉	Vasopressin

(b) Actions of vasopressin

Low blood volume → Brain (Medullary centres) → Stimulation | Inhibition ← Osmoreceptors (Brain)

Kidney tubule ← Vasopressin

Vasopressin receptors in tubule

Water retention → High blood volume

(c) Summary of actions of vasopressin

Actions of vasopressin

Renal (main action)
Increases permeability of luminal collecting duct epithelium to water
Receptor type = V₂
Increases water reabsorption

Cardiovascular
Increases blood pressure by constricting peripheral arterioles, but this effect is lessened by vasopressin's dampening of sympathetic drive
Receptor type = V₁

Clinical scenario

A 23-year-old woman was referred to the Endocrine Clinic complaining of increasing thirst and passing large volumes of urine. She was drinking up to three 2 L bottles of water each day, in addition to tea and coffee. Over the previous 6 months she had started waking at night needing to pass urine and to drink. There was no history of headache, visual impairment, or psychiatric disturbance, no history to suggest pituitary dysfunction and no family history of note. She was taking no medica-

tion. Blood tests showed normal glucose, potassium and calcium levels. Further investigations showed her to have 24-hour urine volume of 4.3 L and serum osmolality of 302 mOsmol/kg with a simultaneous urine osmolality of 276 mOsmol/kg. During a formal water deprivation test, serum osmolality rose with an impaired response of urine osmolality. After intramuscular administration of des-amino-des-aspartate-arginine vasopressin (DDAVP, a long-acting analogue of antidiuretic hormone) her urine promptly concentrated, confirming a diagnosis of cranial diabetes insipidus (DI). She was initially treated with intranasal DDAVP, subsequently converting to oral therapy. Endocrine and radiological investigations of the hypothalamus and pituitary revealed no evidence of a space occupying lesion.

Thirst and polyuria are important clinical symptoms. In the absence of hyperglycaemia, hypercalcaemia and hypokalaemia (all of which produce a secondary nephrogenic DI; Table 35.1) it is important to distinguish between cranial DI, nephrogenic DI and primary (psychogenic) polydipsia.

Biosynthesis

Vasopressin is a nonapeptide, synthesized mainly in nerve terminals in the magnocellular paraventricular and supraoptic neurones of the hypothalamus (Fig. 35a). It is also synthesized in other brain areas. Axons of vasopressin cell bodies project not only to the posterior pituitary, but some also make contact with the fenestrated capillaries of the median eminence portal system, while others project to the spinal cord and other brain centres. Vasopressin biosynthesis is very similar in principle to that of oxytocin, in that it is packaged together with a neurophysin, neurophysin II. The importance of the neurophysins is highlighted by the discovery that in a mutant strain of rats, the 'Brattleboro' rat, a single nucleotide deletion in the second exon of the gene encoding a very highly conserved region of neurophysin II prevents the translation of vasopressin mRNA. These rats suffer from the equivalent of human diabetes insipidus.

Mechanism of action of vasopressin

Vasopressin acts through specific G-protein-coupled receptors on the plasma membrane of the target cell (Fig. 35a). These have been discovered in many organs, including kidney, pituitary, brain, blood vessels, platelets, liver, the gonads and on tumour cells.

Vasopressin receptors. Three subtypes of vasopressin receptors have been discovered V_{1A}, V_{1B} and V_2. The vasopressin V_{1A} receptor mediates glycogenolysis, platelet aggregation, cell proliferation and contraction and release of coagulation factor. Vasopressin receptor V_{1B} is expressed predominantly in the anterior pituitary gland and mediates the release of ACTH, β-endorphin, and prolactin. The vasopressin V_2 receptor is exclusively expressed in the kidney, and defects in this receptor result in nephrogenic diabetes insipidus. V_1 actions are mediated through the IP3 system, whereas V_2 are through cyclic AMP (Fig. 35a).

Physiological actions of vasopressin

Kidney. Vasopressin affects the ability of the renal tubules to reabsorb water (Fig. 35b). The receptors for vasopressin occur principally in the ascending loop of Henle and the collecting ducts, with some in the mesangium (periphery) of the glomerulus. Solutes are powerfully reabsorbed from the loop of Henle, while the walls of the collecting ducts have a variable permeability to water. In the absence of vasopressin, the collecting ducts are impermeable to water, and hypo-osmotic urine is voided. In the chronic state, this is diabetes insipidus. When the plasma concentration of vasopressin is high, for example during dehydration or haemorrhage, the collecting ducts become permeable to water, and hyperosmotic urine is voided, resulting in

Table 35.1 Causes of diabetes insipidus

Cranial	Idiopathic
	Hypothalamic or stalk lesion
	craniopharyngioma, sarcoidosis, head injury, post-pituitary surgery, basal meningitis, shistiocytosis
	Genetic
	Dominant
	Recessive: DIDMOAD syndrome (diabetes insipidus, diabetes mellitus, optic atrophy, deafness)
Nephrogenic	**Primary**
	Genetic: sex-linked recessive, cystinosis
	Secondary
	Metabolic: hyperglycaemia, hypercalcaemia, hypokalaemia
	Drug therapy: lithium, demeclocycline
	Heavy metal poisoning

a concentration of solutes in plasma. In the healthy individual, vasopressin regulates the development of the osmotic gradient as the tubular filtrate passes through the tubules, and ensures the conservation of water by the body. Vasopressin release from the posterior pituitary is determined principally by blood volume. In the hypothalamus, anatomically near to the paraventricular and supraoptic nuclei, there are osmoreceptors, selectively sensitive to sucrose or sodium ions, which are triggered by a rise in the osmolarity of blood. Vasopressin is released and blood volume rises, which switches off osmoreceptor activity.

Blood pressure. Vasopressin is involved in the regulation of blood pressure through its effects on blood volume (Fig. 35c). When this rises, it activates pressure-sensitive receptors in the carotid sinus, the aortic arch and the left atrium, sending afferent messages to the brain stem via the vagus and glossopharangeal nerves, and vasopressin release is inhibited. Vasopressin itself, *within physiological ranges of concentration* in the bloodstream, does not alter blood pressure.

Adrenocorticotrophic hormone (ACTH) and thyroid-stimulating hormone (TSH) secretion are affected by vasopressin, which reaches the anterior pituitary corticotroph via the portal system. It causes ACTH secretion in its own right as a releasing hormone, and also potentiates the action of corticotrophin-releasing factor (see Chapter 18). It is not known, however, how important this effect of vasopressin is in the control of ACTH release. Vasopressin, in physiological concentrations, stimulates the release of TSH from the anterior pituitary thyrotroph, and is equipotent with thyrotrophin-releasing hormone (TRH) in this respect. It has also been discovered that vasopressin actually inhibits TRH release, and it has been suggested that centrally released vasopressin may function in the hypothalamus as part of a 'short-loop' negative-feedback regulator of TSH release.

Liver. Vasopressin has a glycogenolytic action in the liver, where it increases the intracellular concentration of Ca^{2+} in hepatocytes. Vasopressin activates the calcium-dependent phosphorylation of the phosphorylase enzyme that catalyses the conversion of glycogen to glucose phosphate.

Brain. Vasopressin may be involved in memory and male social behaviour.

36 Renin–angiotensin–aldosterone system

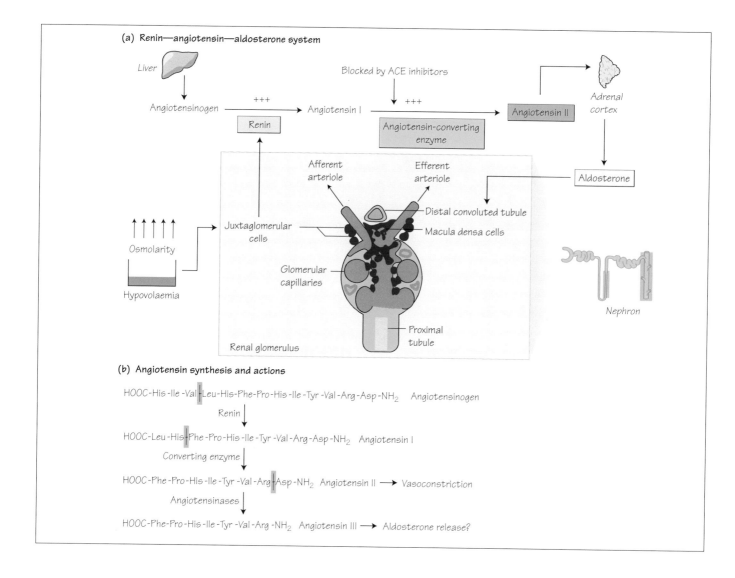

(a) Renin—angiotensin—aldosterone system

Liver

Angiotensinogen →+++→ Angiotensin I →+++→ Angiotensin II → Adrenal cortex

Renin

Blocked by ACE inhibitors

Angiotensin-converting enzyme

Aldosterone

Afferent arteriole

Efferent arteriole

Distal convoluted tubule

Macula densa cells

Juxtaglomerular cells

Osmolarity

Hypovolaemia

Glomerular capillaries

Proximal tubule

Renal glomerulus

Nephron

(b) Angiotensin synthesis and actions

HOOC-His-Ile-Val-Leu-His-Phe-Pro-His-Ile-Tyr-Val-Arg-Asp-NH₂   Angiotensinogen

Renin

HOOC-Leu-His-Phe-Pro-His-Ile-Tyr-Val-Arg-Asp-NH₂   Angiotensin I

Converting enzyme

HOOC-Phe-Pro-His-Ile-Tyr-Val-Arg-Asp-NH₂   Angiotensin II → Vasoconstriction

Angiotensinases

HOOC-Phe-Pro-His-Ile-Tyr-Val-Arg-NH₂   Angiotensin III → Aldosterone release?

Clinical background

Activation of the renin–angiotensin–aldosterone system is an important mechanism in the pathophysiology of heart failure as part of the counter-regulatory neurohormonal response to impaired cardiac output. In conjunction with sympathetic drive, there is an increase in peripheral vasoconstriction mediated by increased sympathetic tone and angiotensin II coupled with the salt and water retention induced by elevated aldosterone concentrations. Together, these increase preload and afterload on the heart, further compromising impaired ventricular function and setting up a vicious circle of heart failure.

Angiotensin–converting enzyme inhibitor drugs (ACE inhibitors) block this increase in aldosterone production and are effective drugs in the clinical management of chronic heart failure. In randomized controlled trials, ACE inhibitors have been shown to improve symptoms and reduce the incidence of further cardiac events including hospital readmission for heart failure, myocardial infarction and death.

Renin

Renin is synthesized and stored in the **juxtaglomerular cells** of the kidney. These are located in the walls of the **afferent arterioles** which supply the glomeruli (Fig. 36a). These arterioles also contain **baroreceptors**, which fire off in response to changes in flow rate and pressure. The cells of the **macula densa** are sensitive to changes in urinary cations such as Ca^{2+}, Na^{2+} and Cl^-. The afferent arterioles, the juxtaglomerular cells and the macula densa are together termed the **juxtaglomerular apparatus**.

Release. Renin is an enzyme with a molecular weight of about 40 kDa which is released in response to a rise in blood osmolarity or to hypovolaemia, although there are different theories as to what the physiological stimuli to release are. The theories are that:

1 the macula densa cells monitor changes in cations and pass this information to the adjacent juxtaglomerular cells;

2 the baroreceptors in the afferent arterioles fire off in response to changes in the mean renal perfusion pressure (the baroreceptors may be part of the juxtaglomerular cells themselves);

3 there is autonomic innervation of juxtaglomerular cells (sympathetic stimulation releases renin).

It is possible that all three theories are significant in the regulation of renin release.

Action. Renin cleaves angiotensinogen to angiotensin I in the plasma and kidney (Fig. 36b). Angiotensinogen is a globulin with a molecular weight of about 60 kDa, which is synthesized continuously in the liver and released in the circulation. Angiotensin I is converted into the biologically active form, the octapeptide **angiotensin II**, by a converting enzyme which occurs in plasma, vascular endothelial cells, kidney, lung and many other tissues. Angiotensin-converting enzyme (ACE) has another function in the inactivation of a potent vasodilator called bradykinin.

Angiotensin II

Angiotensin II is the most potent natural vasoconstrictor so far discovered. The hormone is rapidly inactivated by angiotensinase enzymes in the peripheral capillaries. One of the breakdown metabolites, called **angiotensin III**, occurs in large amounts in the adrenal gland, and has been found to stimulate aldosterone release without significant vasopressor effect. Angiotensin III is a heptapeptide, resulting from the removal of the N-terminal aspartic acid from angiotensin II.

Actions of angiotensin II

1 **Vascular smooth muscle and heart.** Angiotensin II has a potent and direct vasoconstrictor effect on vascular muscle, and plays a critical role in the regulation of arterial blood pressure. There are marked regional differences in constrictor responses to angiotensin II in different vascular beds. Blood vessels in the kidney, mesenteric plexus and the skin are highly responsive to angiotensin II, while those in the brain, lungs and skeletal muscle respond less to administered peptide. In the heart, angiotensin II acts on atrial and ventricular myocytes during the plateau phase of the action potential, to increase Ca^{2+} entry through voltage-gated channels, thereby prolonging the action potential, which increases the force of contraction of the heart.

2 **Kidney.** Angiotensin II regulates glomerular permeability, tubular Na^+ and water reabsorption and renal haemodynamics. Angiotensin II has three important renal actions:

(a) It constricts the renal arterioles, especially the efferent arterioles, which lowers the glomerular filtration rate proportionately more than renal blood flow. This causes an increase in the osmolarity of blood feeding into the peritubular capillaries, which drives solutes and water back into the tubular cell and thence to the bloodstream.

(b) Angiotensin II has been shown to constrict glomerular mesangial cells, which also contributes to the fall in glomerular filtration rate.

(c) Angiotensin II has a direct action on the tubule cells to stimulate Na^+ reabsorption.

3 **Adrenal cortex.** Angiotensin II alone, or through conversion to angiotensin III, acts on the glomerulosa cells to increase aldosterone synthesis.

4 **Nervous system.** Angiotensin II binds to specific presynaptic receptors on sympathetic nerve terminals to enhance norepinephrine release. It has been shown to depolarize adrenal medullary chromaffin cells, causing release of epinephrine, and, when injected directly into the brain, causes an increase in salt and thirst appetite. Angiotensin stimulates vasopressin release from the posterior pituitary gland, an effect potentiated by dehydration.

5 **Water absorption.** Angiotensin II stimulates Na^+ and water absorption from the lumen of the gastrointestinal tract (GIT) at low doses. During dehydration, haemorrhage or salt loss, angiotensin II acts on the small intestine to limit loss, while aldosterone acts predominantly upon the large intestine to limit loss.

6 **Cell proliferation.** Angiotensin II has been shown to have trophic effects on smooth muscle vascular cells, fibroblasts, adrenocortical cells and human fetal kidney mesangial cells. The peptide appears to stimulate the production of specific proteins such as α-actin, and may play a role in repair following vascular injury.

Receptor subtypes. Angiotensin II receptor subtypes have been discovered using different analogues of angiotensin II. The AT_1 receptor, acting through G proteins and the IP3 second messenger system, mediates the increase in blood pressure in extracellular volume and cell proliferation. The AT_2 receptor may mediate cell proliferation.

Tissue distribution of receptor subtypes. Aortic smooth muscle cells, GIT, kidney, liver, lung, placenta and urinary bladder express exclusively AT_1 receptors. Both AT_1 and AT_2 receptors are expressed in the brain, where AT_1 receptors may mediate the central actions of angiotensin II on blood pressure, water and electrolyte balance, the renal arterioles, adrenal cells, heart and uterus. There is evidence for the existence of even more subtypes of angiotensin II receptors.

More recent studies have identified the presence of angiotensin II receptors on the nuclear membrane of cardiomyocytes, which activate NFk ß expression. This suggests a role for angiotensin directly on cardiac function.

37 Endocrine hypertension

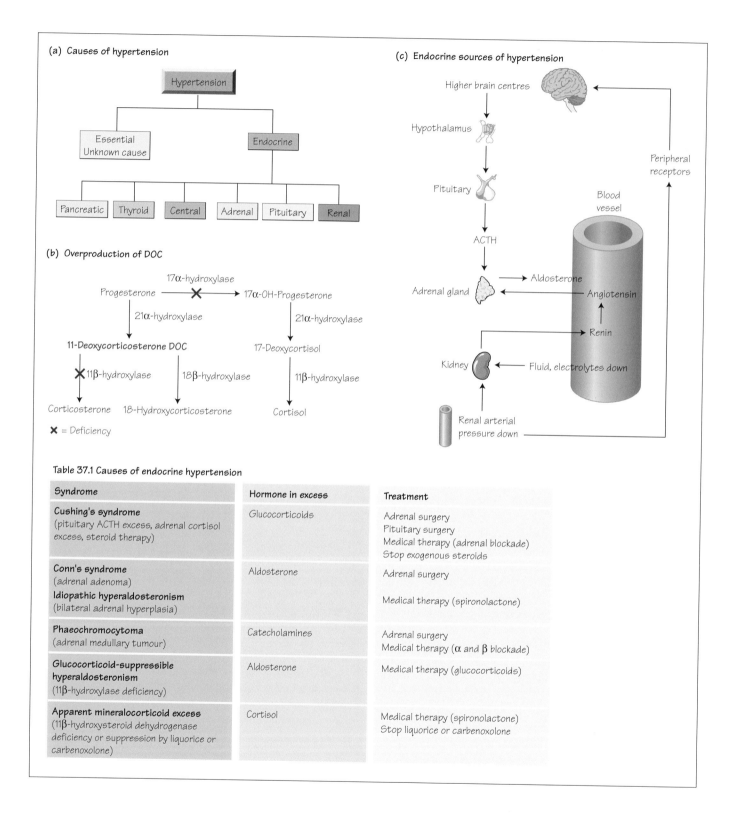

(a) Causes of hypertension

Hypertension

- Essential Unknown cause
- Endocrine
  - Pancreatic
  - Thyroid
  - Central
  - Adrenal
  - Pituitary
  - Renal

(b) Overproduction of DOC

Progesterone — 17α-hydroxylase ✗ → 17α-OH-Progesterone

21α-hydroxylase → 11-Deoxycorticosterone DOC

21α-hydroxylase → 17-Deoxycortisol

11-Deoxycorticosterone DOC:
✗ 11β-hydroxylase → Corticosterone
18β-hydroxylase → 18-Hydroxycorticosterone

17-Deoxycortisol:
11β-hydroxylase → Cortisol

✗ = Deficiency

(c) Endocrine sources of hypertension

Higher brain centres → Hypothalamus → Pituitary → ACTH → Adrenal gland → Aldosterone

Angiotensin

Renin

Blood vessel

Peripheral receptors

Kidney ← Fluid, electrolytes down

Renal arterial pressure down

Table 37.1 Causes of endocrine hypertension

Syndrome	Hormone in excess	Treatment
Cushing's syndrome (pituitary ACTH excess, adrenal cortisol excess, steroid therapy)	Glucocorticoids	Adrenal surgery Pituitary surgery Medical therapy (adrenal blockade) Stop exogenous steroids
Conn's syndrome (adrenal adenoma)	Aldosterone	Adrenal surgery
Idiopathic hyperaldosteronism (bilateral adrenal hyperplasia)		Medical therapy (spironolactone)
Phaeochromocytoma (adrenal medullary tumour)	Catecholamines	Adrenal surgery Medical therapy (α and β blockade)
Glucocorticoid-suppressible hyperaldosteronism (11β-hydroxylase deficiency)	Aldosterone	Medical therapy (glucocorticoids)
Apparent mineralocorticoid excess (11β-hydroxysteroid dehydrogenase deficiency or suppression by liquorice or carbenoxolone)	Cortisol	Medical therapy (spironolactone) Stop liquorice or carbenoxolone

Clinical background

Hypertension affects up to 25% of the population in western countries but only 2–5% will be found to have an identifiable underlying endocrine cause that can be treated. Young people with hypertension should be screened for secondary causes, as should those with a strong family history of hypokalaemia. Treatment is directed towards the underlying cause.

Hypertension may be one of the presenting features of a number of endocrine disorders. Systolic hypertension is typical of thyrotoxicosis, patients with acromegaly are usually hypertensive at presentation and hypertension frequently complicates obesity and diabetes.

Two main types of hypertension are recognized – the first is essential hypertension, which is the most prevalent type and has no known cause but whose aetiology may involve disturbances of endocrine function, particularly the renin–angiotensin–aldosterone system (Fig. 37a). The other is secondary hypertension, which affects around 2–5% of patients, and which is usually the result of endocrine disorders, for example glucocorticoid or catecholamine excess, or hyperaldosteronism.

Clinically, high blood pressure is an important risk factor for cardiovascular diseases such as stroke and myocardial infarction.

Factors raising blood pressure. Blood pressure is raised (i) when the heart beats more powerfully (positive inotropic effect); (ii) when arterioles constrict, increasing the peripheral resistance; (iii) when fluid and salts are retained; and (iv) through the influence of cardiovascular control centres in the brain, or a combination of two or more of these factors.

Hormonal causes of hypertension and treatments
Hypertension of adrenal origin

Phaeochromocytoma (see Chapter 16). Epinephrine, secreted by a phaeochromocytoma (adrenal medullary tumour) raises blood pressure and its effects can be countered using α- and β-blockers and the problem cured by removing the tumour.

Hyperaldosteronism (see Chapter 20). Over-secretion of aldosterone by an adrenal adenoma (**primary hyperaldosteronism; Conn's syndrome**). Aldosterone promotes the retention of Na^+ and water and this expands the plasma volume and raises the blood pressure. This can be treated by blocking aldosterone receptors with spirinolactone and cured by removing the tumour. Aldosterone secretion can also be increased by excess renin secretion, which increases angiotensin II production, which in turn promotes aldosterone release (**secondary hyperaldosteronism**). This mechanism plays an important role in the neurohormonal sequence in heart failure. Secondary hyperaldosteronism can be treated by blocking angiotensin II production with ACE inhibitors, or with angiotensin II receptor antagonists. Aldosterone receptors can also be stimulated through over-production of cortisol or deoxycorticosterone (see below), which bind aldosterone receptors with high affinity. Cortisol is normally rapidly metabolized by 11β-hydroxysteroid dehydrogenase, and patients with an hereditary deficiency or absence of this enzyme exhibit an apparent hyperaldosteronism.

Cushing's disease (see Chapter 17). Raised cortisol concentrations increase angiotensinogen release from the liver. Cortisol, as described above, also stimulates aldosterone receptors.

Excess deoxycorticosterone (DOC) production (Fig. 37b). Clinically, DOC ranks second after aldosterone in importance as a mineralocorticoid. Excess DOC is diagnosed because it reduces renin and aldosterone production by a negative feedback on the latter two hormones. DOC is a potent mineralocorticoid and circulates at about the same concentration as aldosterone. However, DOC is normally inactive because most of it circulates bound to the protein CBG and is inactivated in the liver. Urine is virtually free of DOC. Excess DOC production can occur through overproduction of steroids, as in primary aldosteronism, Cushing's disease (see Chapter 17) or when there are congenital deficiencies of certain steroid-metabolizing enzymes such 11β-hydroxylase which also results in increased androgen production and consequent virilization (see Chapter 19). Congenital deficiency of adrenal 17α-hydroxylase will also promote excess DOC production and consequent hypertension together with impaired sexual maturation in both sexes (see Chapter 19). Deficiencies of 11β-hydroxylase and 17α-hydroxylase are treated with glucocorticoids, which is standard treatment for all forms of congenital adrenal hyperplasia associated with Na^+ retention.

Hypertension of renal origin

The renin–angiotensin–aldosterone system is normally finely tuned through feedback mechanisms to maintain the proper plasma osmolality and K^+ and Na^+ concentrations (Fig. 37c). This balance, together with the integrated operation of the cardiovascular system ensures the maintenance of a healthy blood pressure. This regulatory system may involve the actions of angiotensin in the brain and/or in circumventricular organs of the brain that do not have a blood–brain barrier, for example the area postrema. The precise mechanism is unknown, but it is possible that the brain ultimately regulates renin release from the juxtaglomerular apparatus of the kidney, and a 'resetting' of set points for blood pressure in the brain through the regulation of renin release may be important in the aetiology of essential hypertension (Fig. 37c).

Hypertension of other endocrine origin

Insulin. There is a strong association between hypertension, insulin resistance, hyperinsulinaemia and obesity, and hypertension may be a consequence of the latter three conditions. Indeed, many obese patients with hypertension are also insulin-resistant. In patients with Type 2 diabetes (see Chapter 41), glucose uptake into tissues is impaired with consequent increased insulin release. Insulin stimulates sympathetic activity and promotes Na^+ reuptake in the kidney tubules, and these may contribute to the hypertension produced in these patients.

Thyroid. Hyperthyroidism is associated with systolic hypertension due to a combination of increased cardiac output and reduced peripheral resistance.

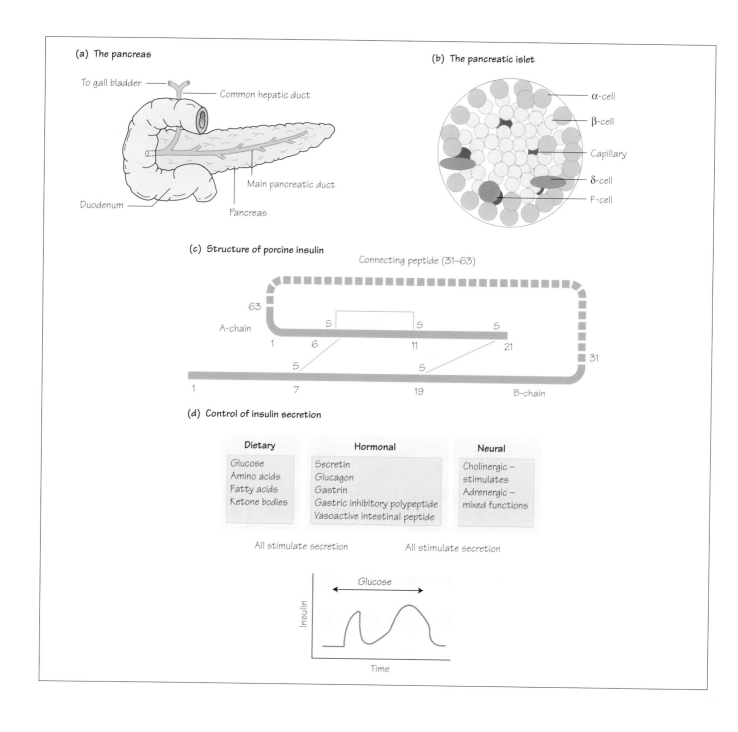

(a) The pancreas

To gall bladder — Common hepatic duct

Main pancreatic duct

Duodenum

Pancreas

(b) The pancreatic islet

α-cell

β-cell

Capillary

δ-cell

F-cell

(c) Structure of porcine insulin

Connecting peptide (31–63)

63

A-chain

1   6   11   21   31

1   7   19   B-chain

(d) Control of insulin secretion

Dietary	Hormonal	Neural
Glucose	Secretin	Cholinergic – stimulates
Amino acids	Glucagon	Adrenergic – mixed functions
Fatty acids	Gastrin	
Ketone bodies	Gastric inhibitory polypeptide	
	Vasoactive intestinal peptide	

All stimulate secretion   All stimulate secretion

Glucose

Insulin

Time

 The Endocrine System at a Glance, 3rd edition. © Ben Greenstein and Diana Wood. Published 2011 by Blackwell Publishing Ltd.

Clinical scenario

A 21-year-old male student, HB, was referred to the Diabetic Clinic of his local hospital. He had been feeling unwell for about 4 weeks, noticing a marked increase in thirst, passage of large volumes of urine both during the day and at night. He felt generally tired and unwell and had lost about 6 kg in weight over the preceding month. Physical examination was normal. A diagnosis of Type 1 diabetes was made on the basis of a random blood glucose of 25 mmol/L and the presence of glucose and ketones in the urine. HB was started on insulin therapy and subsequently managed with a 'basal-bolus' regimen, taking an injection of short-acting insulin 30 minutes before meals and intermediate-acting insulin at bedtime. His symptoms improved over the next few weeks and he attended the clinic for dietary advice and education about testing his own blood glucose, managing hypoglycaemic attacks and monitoring for complications.

Type 1 diabetes is an autoimmune condition causing destruction of the pancreatic β cells (see below). Treatment of Type 1 DM is with insulin, administered as subcutaneous injections by the patient. Therapy is tailored to the individual patient and is commonly given as biphasic insulin containing short and intermediate acting insulins and administered twice daily or as a 'basal-bolus' regimen with intermediate insulin given at bedtime supplemented by short-acting insulin before meals. Patients monitor their blood glucose concentrations using capillary blood glucose testing strips and a portable glucometer.

Glycated haemoglobin reflects diabetic control over a period of weeks to months, reflecting erythrocyte lifespan (120 days) and is used to assess glycaemic control in patients with diabetes. The most commonly reported fraction is haemoglobin A1c (HbA1c), which is increased in diabetes by covalent bonding of glucose. The rate of formation of HbA1c is directly proportional to blood glucose concentrations.

Introduction

The pancreas lies closely adjacent to the duodenum (Fig. 38a) and consists of two major tissue types, namely the acini, which secrete digestive juices into the duodenum, and the islets of Langerhans, which secrete insulin and glucagon directly into the bloodstream, and are therefore truly endocrine. The human pancreas has between 1 and 2 million islets, each organized around small capillaries into which the hormones are secreted. The islet cells can be distinguished into four types: α, β, δ (also called A, B and D) and F (Fig. 38b). The β cells, which constitute about 60% of the islet cells, lie towards the middle of the islet and secrete **insulin**. The α cells secrete **glucagon** and the δ cells secrete **somatostatin**. The other cell type, the F cell, secretes pancreatic polypeptide. A physiological role for pancreatic polypeptide has not yet been identified with certainty.

Insulin

In humans, the gene coding for insulin is located on the short arm of chromosome 11. Insulin is secreted by the β cells of the islets of Langerhans. It is a protein consisting of two chains, an A-chain of 21 amino acids, and a B-chain of 30 amino acids, linked by two disulphide bridges (A7B7 and A20B19; Fig. 38c). Another disulphide bridge links A6A11 on the A-chain. Insulin can exist as a monomer (molecular weight of 6 kDa), the form in which it predominantly circulates. It can dimerize to form a dimer of molecular weight of 12 kDa, and three dimers can aggregate in the presence of two zinc atoms to form a hexamer of molecular weight 36 kDa.

Biosynthesis. Insulin is cleaved from proinsulin. Proinsulin is derived from a larger precursor, preproinsulin, which is synthesized in the rough endoplasmic reticulum. Proinsulin is a continuous chain which starts at the N-terminal end of the B-chain and terminates at the C-terminal end of the A-chain. A connecting peptide (C-peptide; Fig. 38c) is interposed between the C-terminal end of the B-chain and the N-terminal end of the A-chain. In the Golgi apparatus and the storage granules, a converting enzyme cleaves proinsulin to yield insulin.

Secretion of insulin. Insulin synthesis and secretion is stimulated by glucose (Fig. 38d), which stimulates the β cell to take up extracellular calcium (Ca^{2+}). The cation appears to trigger a contractile mechanism, whereby the microtubules participate in the movement of insulin-containing granules towards the cell membrane, where granules fuse and the granule contents are released into the extracellular space by exocytosis. Insulin secretion in response to a sudden rise in circulating glucose occurs in a biphasic fashion: there is an immediate release of stored insulin, lasting less than a minute, followed by a more sustained release of both stored and newly synthesized insulin. A great many other substances stimulate insulin release, but not all elicit a biphasic release pattern. Carbohydrates, most amino acids and, to a lesser extent, fatty acids and ketones, all stimulate insulin release. Although a number of gut hormones can stimulate insulin release, the physiological significance of this, if any, is unknown. Glucagon, which is synthesized in the pancreatic α cells, stimulates insulin release by direct action on the β cells.

Insulin release is also affected by the nervous system and by neurotransmitters. Acetylcholine stimulates insulin release, as does epinephrine, acting on β-receptors. Stimulation of α-receptors, on the other hand, causes an inhibition of insulin release. Stimulation of different areas of the hypothalamus in experimental animals has different effects on insulin release. For example electrical stimulation of the ventrolateral region stimulates insulin release, while electrical stimulation of the ventromedial region inhibits insulin release. The basal secretion of insulin is also affected by neurotransmitters. Drugs which block adrenergic α-receptors increase basal insulin tone, while drugs which block β-receptors reduce basal insulin tone.

Insulin metabolism. Insulin circulates as a monomer, unbound to plasma proteins. It is filtered by the glomeruli, but is almost completely reabsorbed in the proximal tubules, and is degraded by the kidneys. The liver removes half the hepatic portal insulin that passes through it. The half-life of insulin in plasma is about 5 minutes. Proinsulin, which is also released with insulin, has a longer half-life (about 20 minutes). Proinsulin is not cleaved to insulin in the plasma. Although the liver and kidneys are the major sites of insulin degradation, virtually all the tissues of the body can break down the hormone. Insulin can be degraded extracellularly, and also intracellularly, after it has bound to its receptor and become internalized in the cell.

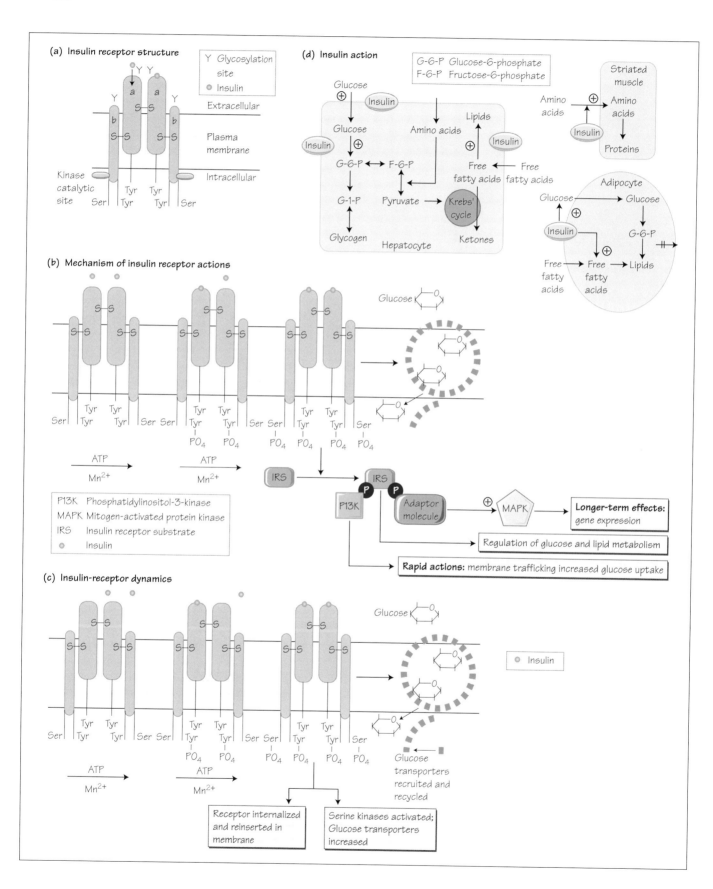

(a) Insulin receptor structure

Y Glycosylation site
○ Insulin

(b) Mechanism of insulin receptor actions

P13K Phosphatidylinositol-3-kinase
MAPK Mitogen-activated protein kinase
IRS Insulin receptor substrate
○ Insulin

(c) Insulin-receptor dynamics

(d) Insulin action

G-6-P Glucose-6-phosphate
F-6-P Fructose-6-phosphate

Longer-term effects: gene expression

Regulation of glucose and lipid metabolism

Rapid actions: membrane trafficking increased glucose uptake

Receptor internalized and reinserted in membrane

Serine kinases activated; Glucose transporters increased

Clinical scenario

Mrs PC, a 45-year-old woman, was referred to her GP having been found to have a raised random blood glucose measurement at an insurance medical examination. On questioning she admitted to feeling increasingly tired recently and her weight had increased over the preceding year. She smoked 15 cigarettes a day. Her mother and maternal grandfather had Type 2 diabetes. On examination she was obese (body mass index $34 \, kg/m^2$). Blood pressure was 160/90 and there was an absent posterior tibial pulse at the right ankle. The rest of the examination was normal. Subsequent investigations revealed a fasting blood glucose of 12.2 mmol/L, HbA1c 9.2%, cholesterol 7.4 mmol/L, normal renal function, glycosuria of 3+ on dipstix urine testing.

She was strongly advised to stop smoking and treatment was commenced with antihypertensives and lipid-lowering agents. She was seen by the specialist nurse and dietician and advised about monitoring her blood glucose and about diet and exercise. Initially, her progress was slow but she eventually started to lose weight after the introduction of the drug metformin. This was accompanied by improved glycaemic control.

Mechanism of action of insulin

The insulin receptor belongs to a superfamily of transmembrane receptor tyrosine kinases. Other members of this receptor superfamily include the receptors for insulin-like growth factor 1 (IGF-1), epidermal growth factor (EGF) and platelet-derived growth factor (PDGF). The insulin receptor consists of subunits: two alpha subunits and two beta subunits, which are linked covalently to each other by disulphide bridges (Fig. 39a). The alpha subunits are extracellular and contain the insulin-binding sites. The beta subunits span the membrane and transduce the binding of insulin to the alpha subunits into an intracellular signal by the following mechanism. When insulin binds to the receptor site, this interaction is transmitted to the intracellular domain of the beta subunit. This subunit becomes autophosphorylated, which in turn activates its own protein kinases, resulting in an intracellular cascade of phosphorylation and dephosphorylation reactions through which the actions of insulin are expressed.

A link between the insulin receptor and the rest of the phosphorylation cascade may be a family of proteins called insulin receptor substrate (IRS). Two IRS proteins, IRS-1 and IRS-2, are essential for the complete expression of the action of insulin. Autophosphorylation of the insulin receptor results in the tyrosine phosphorylation of the IRS proteins. This confers on IRS proteins the ability to bind other sets of signalling proteins that contain signalling domains and this docking process leads, ultimately, to the various effects of insulin on glucose transport, glycogen synthesis, protein synthesis and mitogenesis (Fig. 39b).

Insulin converts glucose into glycogen, and this reaction is controlled by glycogen synthetase, which is inactive in the phosphorylated state, and activated by dephosphorylation. Hepatic phosphorylase, on the other hand, is activated by phosphorylation. Hepatic phosphorylase activates glycogenolysis. It has been suggested that insulin exerts its action on glycogen metabolism through its inhibition of phosphorylation of both these enzymes, possibly through the mechanism involving SH2 domains.

Glucose transporters. Insulin stimulates the cellular uptake of glucose, a major physiological action of insulin. Glucose is taken into the cell by glucose transporters, through a process of facilitated diffusion. The transporters can transfer glucose and other sugars across the cell membrane down a chemical concentration gradient (Fig. 39c). Glucose transporters vary in structure and ionic requirements from tissue to tissue.

Receptor internalization. After the receptor binds insulin, the hormone–receptor complex leaves the membrane through a process of endocytosis and enters the cell. After binding to the receptor, the complex becomes encapsulated in a coated pit, formed by invagination and fusion of the cell surface. Once inside the cell, the pit becomes progressively uncoated to form what is called an endosome. The endosome releases the receptor and insulin, the former being mainly recycled to the membrane, and insulin being degraded. The process of **receptor internalization** may provide a means of regulating the effects of insulin by limiting the numbers of receptors available for binding to the hormone. This mechanism effectively down regulates the insulin receptor.

Insulin effects

After a meal, insulin removes glucose from the circulation and promotes its conversion to glycogen and lipids (Fig. 39d). Insulin promotes the conversion of fatty acids to lipids, and the uptake of amino acids into liver and skeletal muscle, where they are elaborated into protein. Insulin is thus an anabolic hormone.

Liver. The liver is the major site of gluconeogenesis and ketogenesis. Lipid and protein production also take place in the liver. Insulin stimulates a number of enzymes involved in glycogen production, including glycogen synthetase, which catalyses the formation of glycogen. Glycogen is also stored in smaller amounts in skeletal muscle and other cells which need to mobilize energy stores rapidly. Within the cell, glucose is also converted into glucose-6-phosphate, which is unable to leave the cell, since the plasma membrane is impermeable to phosphoric acid esters. This creates a concentration gradient, and more glucose moves into the cell.

Fat. Approximately 90% of stored glucose is as lipids. The adipocyte is therefore an important site of insulin action. Insulin is required for the activation of the enzyme lipoprotein lipase. If insulin is absent, lipoproteins accumulate in the circulation. Insulin also opposes the action of glucagon (see Chapter 42), a hormone which promotes the production of **ketone bodies**. The ketone bodies, acetone, acetoacetic acid and β-hydroxybutyric acid, are an energy source for muscle and brain, especially during prolonged fasting. They are derived from lipids, and are produced in conditions of insulin lack. The ketone bodies inhibit glucose and fatty acid oxidation, which results in the preferential use of the ketone bodies as a source of energy. When their rate of production exceeds their rate of utilization, ketoacidosis will result.

Muscle. Insulin stimulates amino acid uptake into skeletal muscle, and increases the incorporation of amino acids into proteins. These two actions are independent of insulin's action on glucose transport into the cell.

40 Insulin: III Type 1 diabetes mellitus

(a) Insulin lack

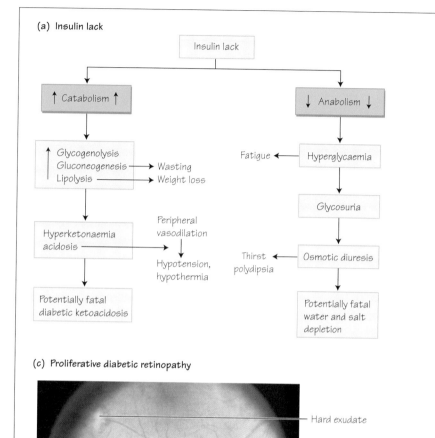

(b) Recommended sites for insulin injection

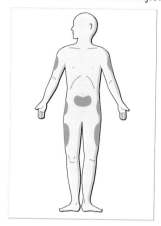

(d) Charcot's arthropathy

Charcot's arthropathy is a more unusual manifestation of diabetic neuropathy in which the joints of the foot become completely disorganized and collapse of the arches of the foot further predisposes to ulceration

(c) Proliferative diabetic retinopathy

Hard exudate

Soft exudate

New vessel formation

Preretinal haemorrhage

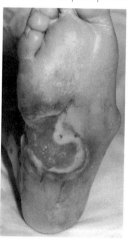

Clinical scenario

Miss GT was a 22-year-old woman with Type 1 diabetes mellitus (DM) since the age of 13. Initially she had been well controlled, but over the last year she had attended her local Accident and Emergency Department on several occasions with hypoglycaemic episodes. For the few days prior to this admission she had felt unwell – she developed an upper respiratory tract infection but despite monitoring her blood sugar more often and taking her insulin, she had started vomiting 8 hours prior to admission. By the time she arrived in the Accident and Emergency Department she was drowsy and had vomited on several further occasions. Her temperature was elevated, she demonstrated prolonged expiration in breathing (Kussmaul's respiration), there was a smell of acetone on her breath and she appeared to be dehydrated and unwell. Her blood glucose was 24 mmol/L and she had both glycosuria and 3+ ketonuria on urinalysis. Blood gases were done immediately and showed a metabolic acidosis with pH 7.2, HCO^3 14 mmol/L, PO^2 12 kPa, PCO^2 3.4 kPa. A diagnosis of diabetic ketoacidosis was made and routine therapy commenced, with IV fluids, potassium and insulin, according to local protocols.

Diabetic ketoacidosis (DKA) is a serious complication of Type 1 DM and presents as a medical emergency. It may be the way in which the disease presents or it may reflect poor compliance with diet and therapy or the effects of a superadded disease such as a chest infection. There is still a significant mortality rate of around 10% associated with DKA and it must be treated seriously, promptly and with meticulous attention to detail in monitoring the response to treatment.

Insulin lack

Insulin lack creates a profoundly catabolic state (Fig. 40a). Without insulin, glucose is not taken up by the tissues, and hyperglycaemia results. The cells are deprived of an energy

Table 40.1 Microvascular complications

Retinopathy	Untreated leading to blindness
Nephropathy	Glomerulosclerosis with progressive proteinuria and renal failure
Neuropathy	Peripheral symmetrical sensory neuropathy – may lead to ulceration and joint collapse in the neuropathic foot
	Charcot's arthropathy (Fig. 40d)
	Mononeuropathies and mononeuritis multiplex including cranial neuropathies
	Amyotrophy (proximal motor neuropathy)
	Autonomic neuropathy – resting tachycardia and postural hypotension; abdominal bloating due to delayed gastric emptying, vomiting and diarrhoea; atonic bladder, erectile dysfunction, gustatory sweating

source and respond by glycogenolysis, gluconeogenesis and lipolysis to generate glucose for energy. This exacerbates the hyperglycaemia, and creates an acidosis through the increased production of ketone bodies, which can prove fatal. The breakdown of body proteins and fats results in weight loss and the acidosis produces vasodilatation and hypothermia. The patient hyperventilates to blow off the acidosis in the form of carbon dioxide. The decreased anabolic state and hyperglycaemia cause fatigue.

Glucose is excreted in the urine, causing excessive diuresis, which in turn results in loss of body fluids and salts. The patient becomes dehydrated, is constantly thirsty and drinks copious volumes of water (polydipsia). Untreated, the patient will eventually fall into a coma, the aetiology of which is not fully understood, but it may result from the combined effects of hyperketonaemia, including dehydration, hyperosmolarity due to hyperglycaemia and problems within the cerebral microcirculation.

Type 1 diabetes mellitus (IDDM)

Type 1 diabetes is an autoimmune condition causing destruction of the pancreatic b cells resulting in absolute insulin deficiency. It presents in children and young adults and is more common in populations of north European origin than other ethnic groups. Infiltration of the pancreatic islets by activated macrophages, cytotoxic and suppressor T lymphocytes and B lymphocytes produces a destructive 'insulitis' which is highly selective for the β cell population. Approximately 70–90% of β cells must be destroyed before the onset of clinical symptoms. Type 1 DM is a polygenic disorder with genetic factors accounting for about 30% of the susceptibility to the disease. There is an association with HLA haplotypes DR3 and DR4 in the major histocompatibility complex on chromosome 6, although these alleles may be markers for other loci responsible for the HLA class II antigens which are involved in initiating the immune response. Environmental factors may also be important in the aetiology of Type 1 diabetes and the role of viruses and diet has been investigated.

Treatment. Patients must take parenteral insulin and follow a carefully regulated diet. Human insulin is now prepared by recombinant DNA technology and is administered by a range of subcutaneous 'pen' devices which simplify insulin delivery. A wide range of insulin preparations are available, ranging from short-acting (soluble), to intermediate-acting to long-acting forms. The aim of treatment is to keep blood glucose levels as close as possible to normal levels, which vary from around 4–9 mmol/L. Patients monitor their own blood glucose regularly throughout the day using a glucometer device and adjust their insulin dosage accordingly. Modern therapy for patients with Type 1 diabetes involves a multidisciplinary approach with doctors, specialist nurses, dieticians, opticians and chiropodists all playing an important role. Patient education is vital to therapy – the more an individual with diabetes understands the condition and is able to regulate their insulin and food intake to their own lifestyle, the better the control and the less likely the onset of serious complications. The DAFNE programme of intensive education related to diet, lifestyle and insulin therapy has proved successful in improving individual's diabetic control. Insulin pump therapy combining real-time glucose monitoring with on-demand insulin therapy offers improved diabetic control to selected patients.

Transplantation of human β-cells. A recent advance is the successful transplantation of human primary islets of Langerhans into patients with Type 1 diabetes. This technique offers hope of a cure, but at the moment the supply of tissue is sparse and the eventual manufacture of islets from stem cells is being investigated.

Poor diabetic control – microvascular complications

All patients with DM should be monitored carefully with the aim of preventing the onset of complications. Patients with Type 1 diabetes are at particular risk of microvascular complications (Table 40.1). Improved glycaemic control reduces the likelihood of developing such complications, particularly diabetic retinopathy (Fig. 40c). Patents should have annual eye checks, preferably with retinal photography combined with direct ophthalmoscopy. The onset of nephropathy is heralded by proteinuria, initially in the form of 'microalbuminuria', that is 30–300 mg/24 h albuminuria. It is important to optimize glycaemic control and blood pressure and ACE inhibitors have been shown to delay progression of microalbuminuria to full blown nephropathy. Neuropathy should be managed by scrupulous foot care including regular chiropody to reduce the likelihood of neuropathic ulcer formation.

Traditionally, microvascular complications were thought to be found exclusively in patients with Type 1 DM. However, improved treatment of cardiovascular disease in patients with Type 2 diabetes means that these complications may be seen in patients with either form of the disease (see Chapter 41).

Islet cells have been generated from murine (mouse) stem cells, which offers hope that this may promise hope for human pancreatic regeneration.

(a) Typical site for pressure ulcer in diabetes, reflecting combined vascular occlusion and neuropathy

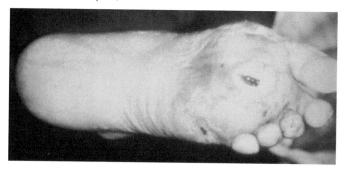

(b) Digital ray ischaemia leading to gangrene with superadded infection

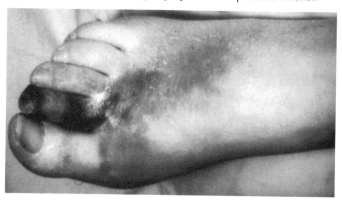

Clinical background

Type 2 diabetes mellitus is a disease that is becoming more common in association with the increase in obesity in the population. The overall UK prevalence is around 2% of the population, rising with age, and is higher in certain ethnic groups including African–Caribbeans (around 5%) and South Asians (>10%). Diagnosis of diabetes depends on the demonstration of a raised non-fasting blood glucose of greater than 11 mmol/L. If there is doubt, a fasting sample should obtained. The guidelines for the diagnosis of DM are shown in Table 41.1. Impaired glucose tolerance is an important condition with a high risk of developing Type 2 DM and an increased risk of macrovascular disease compared to the normal population.

Treatment is of Type 2 diabetes is by dietary measures, lifestyle changes and oral hypoglycaemic agents where necessary. Although patients with Type 2 diabetes do not develop ketosis and do not require insulin for survival, some may be treated with insulin to optimize glycaemic control.

Type 2 diabetes mellitus

Type 2 diabetes mellitus is the most common form of diabetes, accounting for approximately 85% of diabetic patients. It is

Table 41.1 Diagnosis of diabetes mellitus and impaired glucose tolerance (WHO guidelines 1999)

	Venous plasma mmol/L	Venous whole blood mmol/L	Capillary whole blood mmol/L
Diabetes mellitus			
Fasting	≥7.0	≥6.1	≥6.1
2 h postglucose load	≥11.0	≥10.0	≥11.1
Impaired glucose tolerance			
Fasting	<7.0	<6.1	<6.1
2 h postglucose load	≥7.8	≥6.7	≥7.8

characterized by insulin resistance coupled with relative insulin deficiency. The mechanism of insulin resistance in Type 2 diabetes remains unclear. Although numerous genetic abnormalities of the insulin receptor have been identified, in some cases in association with profound insulin resistance syndromes, these are rare and do not explain hyperinsulinaemia seen in the vast majority of patients with Type 2 diabetes. The consequence of prolonged hyperinsulinaemia is the development of insulin deficiency. There is a strong genetic predisposition to Type 2

DM with high levels of concordance between identical twins and high prevalence in certain ethnic communities, particularly individuals of South Asian or African–Caribbean origin. However, environmental factors also play a key role, such that obese individuals have a much higher rate of insulin resistance and Type 2 DM.

Patients may present with symptoms of hyperglycaemia such as thirst and polyuria although more commonly hyperglycaemia is diagnosed during routine investigations or in patients with cardiovascular disease, urinary tract or skin infections. Investigations reveal elevated blood glucose and glycated haemoglobin concentrations, usually associated with dyslipidaemia. Residual insulin secretion means that individuals with Type 2 diabetes do not develop ketoacidosis, although they may present as an emergency with hyperosmolar non-ketotic coma (HONK) induced by prolonged hyperglycaemia and subsequent dehydration and hypernatraemia. These patients require careful management with fluid replacement and small doses of insulin to restore euvolaemia and euglycaemia prior to establishment on diet and oral hypoglycaemic therapy.

Historically, Type 2 diabetes has occurred more commonly in patients over the age of 40 years. However, with the rising incidence of obesity in western populations and its earlier onset, it is now encountered with increasing frequency in young adults and children.

Treatment of Type 2 diabetes

The primary objective is to control plasma levels of glucose and lipids and to lower blood pressure if it is raised. Patients should be encouraged to lose weight and give up smoking, since these are additional risk factors for hypertension and cardiovascular disease, both more common in Type 2 diabetes.

Initially, dietary advice is given. The aim is to achieve normal blood glucose concentrations with control of hyperlipidaemia and blood pressure. Seventy-five per cent of these patients will be overweight or obese and initially the treatment of choice is diet, which aims to reduce the patient's weight to the ideal level. When an appropriate weight for the patient has been achieved, the diet may be adjusted to maintain it at the desired level. Regular exercise, tailored to the patient's abilities, should be encouraged as this helps to increases insulin sensitivity and reduce blood glucose levels. If lipid levels and blood pressure are not controlled then the early introduction of lipid-lowering therapies, usually in the form of statins and antihypertensives, is required. In the absence of good glycaemic control by dietary measures, oral hypoglycaemics are introduced. Initial therapy is usually in the form of sulphonylureas, such as gliclazide or glipizide, which promote insulin secretion, or the biguanide metformin which alters peripheral glucose metabolism. Newer therapies may be added, such as the thiazolidinediones, which reduce peripheral insulin resistance, and acarbose, which inhibits α-glucosidase and lowers postprandial glucose concentrations. Insulin may be required to achieve good glycaemic control in patients with Type 2 diabetes when there has been prolonged poor control and/or symptoms of insulin deficiency supervene.

Clinical management of Type 2 diabetes requires a multidisciplinary approach.

Table 41.2 Macrovascular complications of diabetes

Cardiovascular disease
  Increased prevalence of hypertension
  Ischaemic heart disease associated with abnormal lipid profiles
    leading to myocardial infarction, heart failure
  Hyperglycaemia accelerates the progression of atherosclerosis
Cerebrovascular disease
  Stroke
Peripheral vascular disease
  Intermittent claudication
  Gangrene
  Diabetic foot problems – ischaemia and ulceration

Gestational diabetes. Patients with a predisposition to Type 2 diabetes may present during pregnancy, usually with asymptomatic hyperglycaemia diagnosed routinely. It is vital to achieve excellent glycaemic control to prevent complications in the newborn and these subjects require detailed monitoring and insulin therapy, sometimes in large doses. Unless diet and lifestyle changes are introduced after the pregnancy a high percentage (>75%) of these women will go on to develop Type 2 diabetes in later life.

Macrovascular complications are the major cause of death in people with Type 2 diabetes, accounting for 50% of deaths in this group (Table 41.2). The relative risk for cardiovascular disease is two to three times higher in men and three to four times higher in women with diabetes than age-matched controls. Diabetics are three times more likely to have a stroke and 15 times more likely to undergo lower limb amputation than non-diabetic subjects. In the long term, patients with Type 2 diabetes may also develop microvascular complications such that diabetic nephropathy is now the second most common cause of end-stage renal disease in the UK.

The diabetic foot

Foot disease in diabetics may be caused by peripheral vascular disease or by neuropathy but commonly there is an element of both (Figs 41a and b). Impaired vascular supply coupled with external pressure from shoes or at pressure points predisposes to tissue necrosis and the formation of ischaemic ulcers and digital gangrene. Ischaemic feet are characterized by weak or absent pulses, pale, cool skin and poor capillary return. Peripheral neuropathy causes weakness of the dorsal interossei muscles allowing unopposed action of the long flexors in the foot and subsequent clawing of the toes. There is a redistribution of pressure throughout the foot allowing ulceration to develop over the metatarsal heads. The loss of pain and joint position sensation contributes to the problem as external irritants (such as stones in the shoes) may go unnoticed by the patient, leading to breakdown of the skin and the onset of ulceration. Neuropathic feet are warm with bounding pulses and dry skin.

Management of foot disease in diabetes is critical to maintaining mobility and prevention of ulceration, gangrene and possible amputation.

42 Glucagon

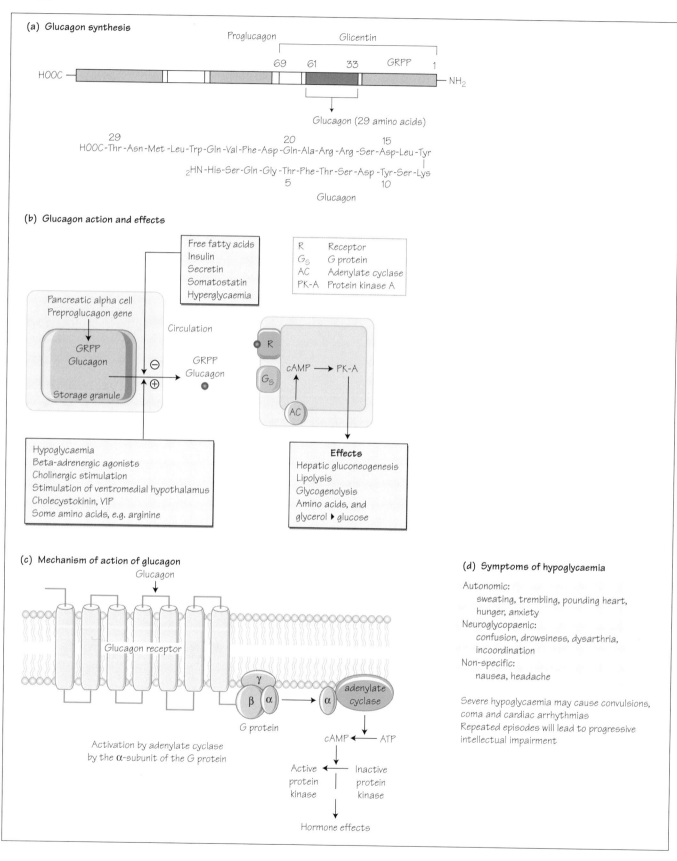

(a) Glucagon synthesis

Proglucagon

Glicentin

HOOC — ... 69 61 33 GRPP 1 — NH₂

Glucagon (29 amino acids)

29
HOOC-Thr-Asn-Met-Leu-Trp-Gln-Val-Phe-Asp-Gln-Ala-Arg-Arg-Ser-Asp-Leu-Tyr
20   15
₂HN-His-Ser-Gln-Gly-Thr-Phe-Thr-Ser-Asp-Tyr-Ser-Lys
5   10

Glucagon

(b) Glucagon action and effects

Free fatty acids
Insulin
Secretin
Somatostatin
Hyperglycaemia

R   Receptor
G_S   G protein
AC   Adenylate cyclase
PK-A   Protein kinase A

Pancreatic alpha cell
Preproglucagon gene

Circulation

GRPP
Glucagon

Storage granule

⊖
⊕

GRPP
Glucagon

R

G_S

cAMP → PK-A

AC

Hypoglycaemia
Beta-adrenergic agonists
Cholinergic stimulation
Stimulation of ventromedial hypothalamus
Cholecystokinin, VIP
Some amino acids, e.g. arginine

Effects
Hepatic gluconeogenesis
Lipolysis
Glycogenolysis
Amino acids, and
glycerol ▶ glucose

(c) Mechanism of action of glucagon

Glucagon

Glucagon receptor

γ
β α

G protein

α

adenylate
cyclase

Activation by adenylate cyclase
by the α-subunit of the G protein

cAMP ◀ ATP

Active ◀ Inactive
protein   protein
kinase   kinase

Hormone effects

(d) Symptoms of hypoglycaemia

Autonomic:
   sweating, trembling, pounding heart,
   hunger, anxiety
Neuroglycopaenic:
   confusion, drowsiness, dysarthria,
   incoordination
Non-specific:
   nausea, headache

Severe hypoglycaemia may cause convulsions,
coma and cardiac arrhythmias
Repeated episodes will lead to progressive
intellectual impairment

Clinical background

Hypoglycaemia is an important complication of insulin therapy in patients with diabetes. At the onset of the disease most patients recognize the symptoms (Fig. 42d) and are able to take remedial action, but 'hypoglycaemia awareness' decreases with the duration of insulin treatment so that after 20 years of diabetes up to a half of patients may have lost their awareness of the symptoms.

Severe hypoglycaemia, requiring the assistance of another person for treatment, is an important cause of morbidity and mortality in insulin treated diabetics. Family members, friends or school staff should be educated in recognition of the symptoms and how to treat it. Early symptoms can be treated with oral carbohydrate; if the patient is unable to swallow intramuscular glucagon is helpful as is buccal glucose gel. Patients and their relatives can be trained to administer intramuscular glucagon. If there is evidence of impaired consciousness medical advice should be sought and the patient treated with intravenous glucose.

Biosynthesis, storage and secretion

Glucagon is synthesized principally in the pancreatic α-cell, and is cleaved from a much larger precursor molecule, preproglucagon (179 amino acids in humans). The preproglucagon gene in humans is located on chromosome 2. Preproglucagon yields proglucagon (Fig. 42a). The N-terminal fragment of proglucagon is termed glicentin-related polypeptide fragment (GRPP), so-called because it contains glicentin (glucagon-like immunoreactivity-1), an intestinal glucagon sequence-containing polypeptide. GRPP and glucagon are stored together in the cell in granules, and released together in approximately equimolar quantities.

Both these peptides are also stored and released from cells in the gut, and glucagon and GRPP form part of a larger family of gut hormones (see Chapter 43). The glucagon content of a healthy human adult pancreas ranges from about 3–5 μg/g of net pancreas weight.

Chemically, glucagon is a polypeptide of molecular weight of about 3.5 kDa, consisting of 29 amino acids. The amino acid sequence of glucagon has been well conserved throughout evolution, and the whole amino acid sequence is required for full biological activity. If the N-terminal histidine is replaced, the molecule loses biological activity. Insulin, on the other hand, depends for its action more on the integrity of its three-dimensional structure, rather than an absolute dependence on the amino acid sequence. Unlike insulin, glucagon does not have a stable three-dimensional structure in physiological solutions, but may acquire this when it binds to its receptor.

Secretion of glucagon (Fig. 42b). Glucagon is rapidly secreted when plasma glucose concentrations fall, and secretion is inhibited when glucose concentrations rise. Secretion is inhibited also by other energy substrates, such as ketone bodies and fatty acids. Amino acids, particularly arginine, stimulate glucagon secretion (as they do insulin). In this situation, where both insulin and glucagon are released simultaneously, the effect may be to allow insulin to promote protein synthesis without a disturbance of normal glucose homeostasis.

Insulin inhibits glucagon secretion (Fig. 42b), perhaps through a paracrine reciprocal interaction between the pancreatic α and β cells. Glucagon secretion is affected by gut hormones (see Chapter 43), being stimulated by cholecystokinin (CCK) and vasointestinal peptide (VIP). Somatostatin, another hormone secreted by the pancreas, among many other tissues, inhibits the secretion of both glucagon and insulin.

The nervous system mediates glucagon release, which is effected by cholinergic and β-adrenergic stimulation. Electrical stimulation of the ventromedial hypothalamus in experimental animals increases glucagon release.

Once released into the circulation, glucagon circulates unbound to any plasma protein, and exists in several forms. The hormone has a short half-life of about 5 minutes, being rapidly degraded, especially in the kidney and liver. In the liver, glucagon binds to a specific membrane receptor, after which it is degraded, a degradation process apparently peculiar to glucagon.

Mechanism of action

Glucagon binds to a membrane receptor on the target cell and activates the adenylate cyclase second messenger system (Fig. 42c). It was through the study of glucagon action on gluconeogenesis that the second messenger system of cellular response was first discovered. Glucose up-regulates glucagon receptor expression while glucagon and agents that increase intracellular cAMP down-regulate glucagon receptor expression. **Glucagon receptor antagonists have now been identified and may become available for controlling circulating glucose in patients.**

Effects of glucagon

Glucagon has the opposite effects to those exerted by insulin. In the **liver**, the hormone promotes the formation of glucose from the breakdown of glycogen. Glucagon, through cAMP, blocks the enzyme cascade leading to glycogen synthesis at the level of the enzyme activities between fructose-6-phosphate and fructose-1,6-diphosphate, and between pyruvate and phosphoenolpyruvate. The glycolytic action of glucagon is essential for maintaining short-term glucose blood levels, especially in the fed state, when glycogen stores are high. In the liver, glucagon promotes the conversion of amino acids to glucose. The hormone also promotes the conversion of free fatty acids to ketone bodies.

Within the **hepatocyte**, glucagon is lipolytic, liberating free fatty acids and glycerol, but its actions on the hepatocyte may only be significant when insulin concentrations are low, since insulin is a potent inhibitor of hepatocyte lipolysis.

Glucagon receptor mutations

Like mutations in the insulin receptor, mutations in the glucagon receptor gene have been reported to be linked to Type 2 diabetes. A single heterozygous missense mutation in exon 2 of the glucagon receptor gene, which changes a glycine to a serine (Gly40Ser), was associated with diabetes in a population of patients with Type 2 diabetes. The mutated receptor was studied *in vitro* and the mutant receptor bound glucagon with an approximately three-fold lower affinity compared with the wild type receptor. Furthermore, the production of cAMP in response to glucagon was decreased in cells expressing the mutant receptor compared with those expressing the wild type.

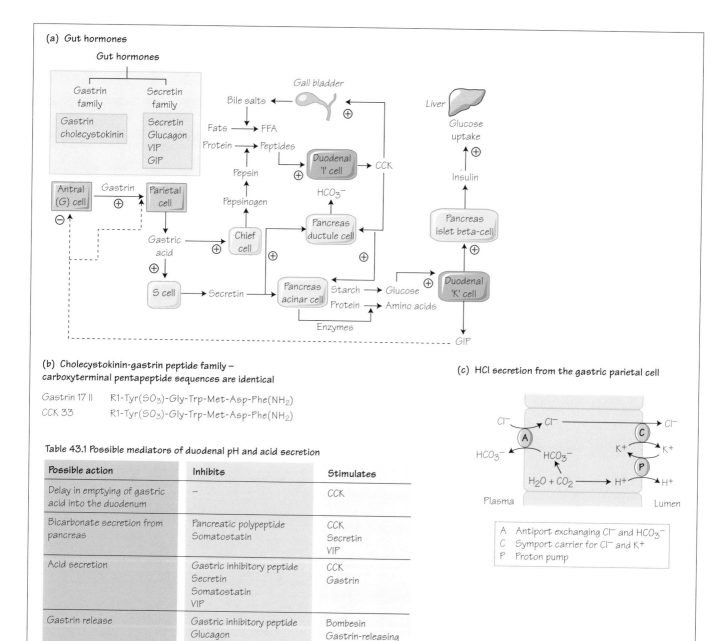

(a) Gut hormones

(b) Cholecystokinin-gastrin peptide family –
carboxyterminal pentapeptide sequences are identical

Gastrin 17 II   R1-Tyr(SO₃)-Gly-Trp-Met-Asp-Phe(NH₂)
CCK 33   R1-Tyr(SO₃)-Gly-Trp-Met-Asp-Phe(NH₂)

(c) HCl secretion from the gastric parietal cell

A   Antiport exchanging Cl^- and HCO_3^-
C   Symport carrier for Cl^- and K^+
P   Proton pump

Table 43.1 Possible mediators of duodenal pH and acid secretion

Possible action	Inhibits	Stimulates
Delay in emptying of gastric acid into the duodenum	–	CCK
Bicarbonate secretion from pancreas	Pancreatic polypeptide Somatostatin	CCK Secretin VIP
Acid secretion	Gastric inhibitory peptide Secretin Somatostatin VIP	CCK Gastrin
Gastrin release	Gastric inhibitory peptide Glucagon Secretin Somatostatin VIP	Bombesin Gastrin-releasing peptide (GRP)

Clinical background

Neuroendocrine tumours of the gastrointestinal system are rare tumours that usually present with manifestations related to the actions of the peptide that they secrete. Functioning neuroendocrine tumours include: the pancreatic tumours insulinomas (insulin secreting), VIPomas (vasoactive intestinal polypeptide), glucagonomas (glucagon), gastrinomas (gastrin) and somatostatinomas (somatostatin) and the small bowel tumours carcinoids (5HIAA), gastrinomas (gastrin) and somatostatinomas (somatostatin). Pancreatic tumours may form part of the MEN 1 syndrome and sometimes secrete a number of other hormones including ACTH (presenting as Cushing's syndrome), GHRH (causing acromegaly), and PTHrP (presenting with hypercalcaemia). Patients with insulinomas present with hypoglycaemic symptoms; those with gastrinomas have complex peptic ulcer disease with diarrhoea; VIPomas cause diarrhoea, acid–base disturbances and glucose intolerance and an erythematous rash; glucagonomas cause a typical necrolytic skin lesion associated with glucose intolerance, bowel disturbance, neuropsychiatric problems and venous thrombosis;

and somatostatinomas present with steatorrhoea, gallstones and diabetes. Carcinoid tumours are the most common of the group, presenting with flushing, diarrhoea, bronchospasm, arthropathy and cardiac complications. All these tumours are extremely rare and require specialist management by multidisciplinary teams of endocrinologists, surgeons, radiologists and oncologists.

Introduction

Gastrointestinal endocrine hormones are principally peptides. Many peptides are synthesized by GIT cells but their role as hormones is unclear. The GIT hormones release enzymes necessary for digestion; they enhance enzyme activity by stimulating the release of bile acids, which provide an optimal acid pH for many enzymes, and the bile salts; some alter GIT motility. Possible mediators of acid secretion and duodenal pH control are shown in Table 43.1.

Biosynthesis, chemistry and release

The GIT hormones are synthesized in 'clear' cells, named because of their selective staining with silver salts, and are widely diffused throughout the gut, thus giving rise to the DES, or **diffuse endocrine system** of the gut. Gut cells have been arbitrarily named, for example G cells (gastrin-secreting), S cells (secretin-secreting), D cells (somatostatin-secreting), K cells (gastric inhibitory peptide-secreting) and I cells (cholecystokinin-secreting). The GIT hormones are conveniently grouped according to their structural similarities into two main families – the **gastrin** and **secretin** families (Fig. 43a).

The secretin family of peptides, namely secretin, glucagon, VIP and gastric inhibitory peptide (GIP) share sequence homology in many amino acids. Secretin and glucagon have 14 amino acids in common. The gastrin family is so-called because gastrin and cholecystokinin (CCK) have identical C-terminal sequences of the first five amino acids (Fig. 43b).

Gastrin is secreted by the G cells in the gastric antrum and the duodenum, and exists in the circulation in several forms, the major ones being G17 and G34, representing the numbers of amino acids in each. G17 is found in the stomach and G34 mainly in the duodenum, and, in humans, in the circulation. The main physiological actions of gastrin are to release HCl from the parietal cells of the stomach (Fig. 43a), and to regulate growth of the gastric mucosa. The acidic gastric juice produced by gastrin excites pepsinogen secretion from the chief cells and secretin release from the S cell. Gastrin release is stimulated mainly by food and to a lesser extent by free fatty acids, amino acids and peptides, but dietary sugars do not release gastrin. The hormone is also released following autonomic vagal stimulation. Gastrin increases motor activity in the GIT, stimulates enzyme secretion from the pancreas, relaxes the pyloric sphincter and increases lower oesophageal sphincter pressure. The mechanism of HCL release from the gastric parietal cell is shown in Fig. 43c.

Cholecystokinin (CCK). CCK-secreting cells (I-cells) occur mainly in the duodenum and the proximal jejunum. CCK has also been described in neurones innervating the distal intestine. In the GIT, CCK is released in response to certain amino acids, particularly tryptophan and phenylalanine, lipids and free fatty acids. CCK contracts the gall bladder and stimulates the release of pancreatic enzymes. CCK stimulates glucagon release, as does VIP. CCK enhances the action of secretin in stimulating bicarbonate release from the pancreas, and it delays gastric emptying. CCK, or a related peptide, may serve as a satiety hormone.

Secretin. In humans, secretin is found predominantly in the granular S cells in the villi and crypts of the small intestinal mucosa. Secretin is released in response to acidification of the contents of the duodenum, that is the entry of gastric fluids. Secretin is not released above a pH of 4.5. Its major action is to stimulate bicarbonate secretion from the pancreas, and it potentiates CCK-invoked release of pancreatic enzymes. Clearly, there is a negative-feedback relationship between secretin and bicarbonate which inhibits secretin release.

Vasointestinal peptide (VIP). Human VIP is a strongly basic polypeptide of 28 amino acids, belonging to the secretin family of peptides. VIP is widely distributed throughout the body, but especially in the GIT, where it occurs from oesophagus to rectum. VIP-containing neurones are especially concentrated in the jejunum, ileum, colon, gall bladder wall, the sphincters and the pancreas. VIP release from cells is known to be modified by other neurones, which contain opioids or somatostatin as neurotransmitters. An important function of VIP within the gut may be to promote descending relaxation, as it is released only during relaxation.

Gastric inhibitory peptide (GIP) is a 42 amino acid polypeptide of the secretin family, present in the GIT at highest concentrations in the duodenum and jejunum. GIP release is stimulated by glucose, amino acids and free fatty acids, and release may also be modified by other hormones. An important action of GIP is to enhance insulin secretion under conditions of hyperglycaemia. Glucose taken orally is more potent in stimulating insulin release than when taken intravenously, and this may be explained by the stimulant effect of glucose on GIP release.

Gastrin-releasing peptide (GRP) is a 27 amino acid (porcine) peptide present in the brain and GIT neurones. GRP, when introduced into rat brain, causes gastrin release from the G cell. GRP has been localized to nerve cells in the antral mucosa, and has been shown to produce a release of gastrin.

Enteroglucagon is the name given to a heterogeneous group of peptides within the gut. These are fragments of the proglucagon molecule, and include a peptide termed oxyntomodulin, and glicentin and GRP. The highest concentrations occur in the ileum and colon, and about 60–80% of the activity is accounted for by glicentin. The peptides are released by food in the gut, which is not the stimulus for glucagon release.

Ghrelin is a peptide hormone synthesized and released from the fundus of the stomach. Ghrelin potently stimulates growth hormone release from the pituitary. It is also orexigenic (promotes feeding behaviour) through an action in the hypothalamus (see also Chapter 45) and is therefore part of the energy balance system.

Motilin is a peptide secreted in the small intestine and is chemically unrelated to other known GIT hormones. Motilin causes periodic contractions of the muscles of the upper GIT, and may perform 'housekeeping' duties to keep the GIT free of undigested material.

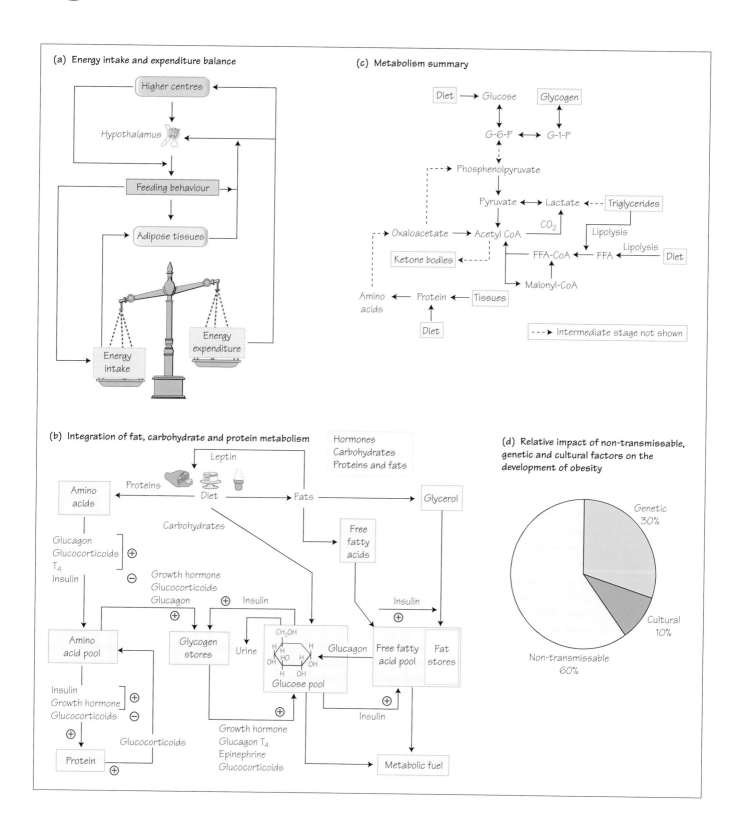

(a) Energy intake and expenditure balance

(c) Metabolism summary

(b) Integration of fat, carbohydrate and protein metabolism

(d) Relative impact of non-transmissable, genetic and cultural factors on the development of obesity

Clinical background

In recent years, adipose tissue has become recognized as a highly metabolically active organ. In 1994, the hormone leptin was identified, a peptide almost exclusively secreted by adipose cells and with receptors both in the hypothalamus and peripheral tissues. Leptin has a number of actions both in relation to signalling satiety and altering energy metabolism. The identification of a rare family with leptin deficiency, extreme obesity and insulin resistance was followed by treatment of two children with recombinant leptin and successful loss of weight. However, in the majority of non-leptin-deficient obese individuals, circulating leptin levels are high and correlated with body fat mass, suggesting that leptin resistance may play a role in human obesity. Further work is needed to establish the exact role of this hormone in energy homeostasis.

Endocrine hormones and energy metabolism

The neuroendocrine system plays a critical role in energy metabolism and homeostasis and is implicated in the control of feeding behaviour. Energy metabolism centres on the maintenance of an adequate supply of glucose for metabolism and on the balance between energy storage and utilization (Fig. 44a). The rapid spread of obesity, with attendant diabetes and heart disease, in western affluent societies has promoted research that has identified previously unknown endocrine hormones that regulate, and indeed dictate, feeding behaviour in other species (see below and Chapter 45).

Energy stores

Fats are the main energy stores in the body. Fats provide the most efficient means of storing energy in terms of kJ/g, and the body can store seemingly unlimited amounts of fat, a fact evident from the phenomenon of extreme obesity. Carbohydrate constitutes <1% of energy stores, and tissues such as the brain are absolutely dependent on a constant supply of glucose, which must be supplied in the diet or by gluconeogenesis. Proteins contain about 20% of the body's energy stores, but since proteins have a structural and functional role, their integrity is defended, except in fasting, and these stores are therefore not readily available.

Circulating glucose can be considered as a **glucose pool** (Fig. 44b), which is in a dynamic state of equilibrium, balancing the inflow and outflow of glucose. The sources of inflow are the diet (carbohydrates) and hepatic glycogenolysis. The outflows are to the tissues, for glycogen synthesis, for energy use, or, if plasma concentrations reach a sufficient level, into the urine. This level is not usually reached in normal, healthy people.

Regulation of the glucose flows is through the action of endocrine hormones, these being epinephrine, growth hormone, insulin, glucagon, glucocorticoids and thyroxine. Insulin is the only hormone with a hypoglycaemic action, whereas all the others are hyperglycaemic, since they stimulate glycogenolysis. Thus, falling blood glucose stimulates their release, while raised glucose stimulates insulin release, an example of dual negative-feedback control.

Integration of fat, carbohydrate and protein metabolism is essential for the effective control of the glucose pool. Two other pools are drawn upon for this, these being the free fatty acid (FFA) pool and the amino acid (AA) pool (Fig. 44b). The FFA pool comprises the balance between dietary FFA absorbed from the GIT, FFA released from adipose tissue after lipolysis, and FFA entering the metabolic process. Insulin drives FFA into storage as lipids, while glucagon, growth hormone and epinephrine stimulate lipolysis. The AA pool in the bloodstream comprises the balance between protein synthesis and the entry of amino acids into the gluconeogenic pathways. A summary of metabolism is shown in Fig. 44c.

Endocrine control of food intake

The discovery of the hormone leptin, which is secreted from adipose tissue and which inhibits feeding behaviour in rodents, has stimulated an interest in the role of the neuroendocrine system in feeding behaviour and the occurrence of obesity. There is now evidence for a feedback system in the hypothalamus (see Chapter 45). In humans, food intake is determined by a number of factors, including the peripheral balance between usage and storage of energy, and by the brain, which through its appetite and satiety centres can trigger and terminate feeding behaviour (Fig. 44a). Leptin is secreted by human adipocytes but it may be more important (in the human) in the long-term maintenance of adequate energy stores during periods of energy deficit, rather than as a short-term satiety hormone.

Feeding behaviour in humans can be initiated and sustained not only through hunger, but also through an awareness of the availability of especially palatable foods and by emotional states; the central mechanisms underlying this behaviour are poorly understood. Conversely, feeding behaviour can be deliberately suppressed, as in anorexia nervosa, when the patient fasts regardless of the knowledge of the consequence of this behaviour. There is, however, a growing body of evidence that in some families there may be genetic contributions, for example mutations of the gene that expresses the melanocortin-4 receptor (MCR-4) gene has been described in rare families with obesity in which satiety is not recognized. The relative contributions of cultural, genetic and non-transmissible factors in the development of obesity are shown in Fig. 44d.

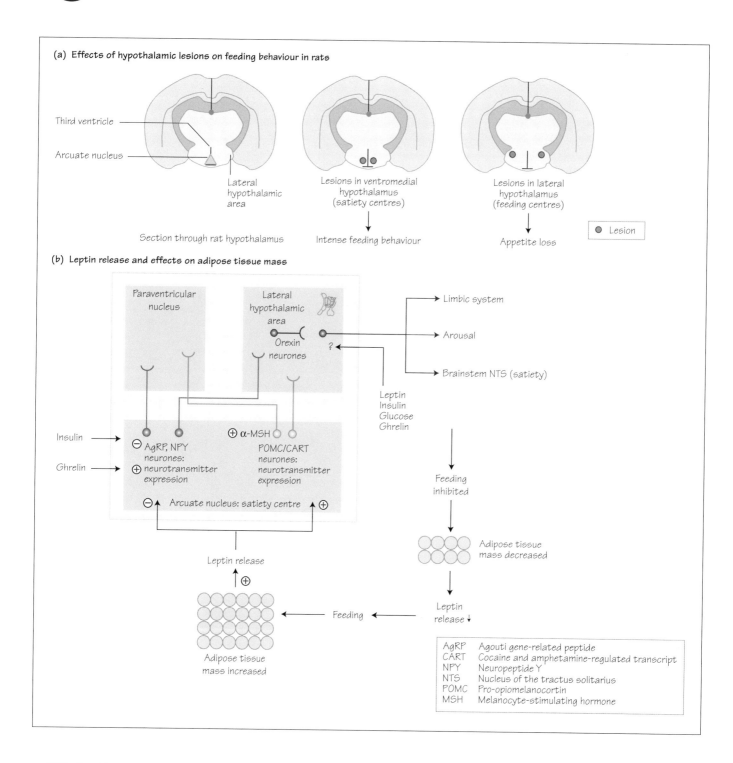

(a) Effects of hypothalamic lesions on feeding behaviour in rats

Third ventricle

Arcuate nucleus

Lateral hypothalamic area

Section through rat hypothalamus

Lesions in ventromedial hypothalamus (satiety centres)

Intense feeding behaviour

Lesions in lateral hypothalamus (feeding centres)

Appetite loss

● Lesion

(b) Leptin release and effects on adipose tissue mass

Paraventricular nucleus

Lateral hypothalamic area

Orexin neurones

→ Limbic system

→ Arousal

? ←

→ Brainstem NTS (satiety)

Leptin
Insulin
Glucose
Ghrelin

Insulin →

Ghrelin →

⊖ AgRP, NPY neurones:
⊕ neurotransmitter expression

⊕ α-MSH

POMC/CART neurones:
neurotransmitter expression

⊖ ▲ Arcuate nucleus: satiety centre ⊕

Leptin release
⊕

Adipose tissue mass increased

Feeding ←

Feeding inhibited

Adipose tissue mass decreased

Leptin release ↓

AgRP	Agouti gene-related peptide
CART	Cocaine and amphetamine-regulated transcript
NPY	Neuropeptide Y
NTS	Nucleus of the tractus solitarius
POMC	Pro-opiomelanocortin
MSH	Melanocyte-stimulating hormone

Clinical scenario

PG, a 15-year-old boy, presented to the paediatric endocrine clinic with delayed puberty and complaining of thirst and polyuria. Investigations revealed hypopituitarism and diabetes insipidus caused by a craniopharyngioma, a cystic tumour of the hypothalamus. He was treated with surgery and radiotherapy. Postoperatively he had deficiencies of all the anterior pituitary hormones requiring hormone replacement and persistent diabetes insipidus treated with DDAVP (see Chapter 35). In the year following treatment he gained 22 kg in weight. He found it extremely difficult to control his food intake and his mother noticed he would continue to eat any food that was in front of him. Attempts to follow a calorie-restricted diet failed.

Energy homeostasis is controlled by the integration of autonomic input and peripheral signals by the brain. Hypothalamic regions involved in this process have been identified in experimental systems, predominantly involving two neuronal populations, the orexigenic neuropeptide Y/Agouti-related peptide neurones and the anorexic pro-opiomelanocortin/ cocaine and amphetamine-related transcript (CART) system. These are interconnected and affected by a number of hormones including insulin, glucocorticoids and leptin. It is likely that the hypothalamic obesity syndrome seen in patients with diseases of the hypothalamus and suprasellar regions relates to disruption of these homeostatic mechanisms.

Introduction

Several lines of evidence point to an important neural role in the control of energy homeostasis, whose status depends mainly on the synchronization of food intake, energy utilization and energy storage. This synchronization appears to be effected largely by the autonomic and neuroendocrine systems. Lesions in the lateral hypothalamus block feeding behaviour in rats to the point of starvation, while lesions in the ventromedial area cause voracious feeding and massively obese rats (Fig. 45a). Humoral signals from the GIT, for example, CCK, or insulin from the pancreas, or glucocorticoids from the adrenal gland, are orexigenic, that is they promote feeding behaviour, while certain hypothalamic hormones, for example TRH and CRH are anorexigenic. The satiety hormone leptin, which is secreted by adipose cells, is an important mediator of the balance between food intake and energy expenditure and conservation. The hypothalamus monitors its blood levels and adjusts feeding behaviour accordingly.

Central regulation of feeding behaviour

The **arcuate nucleus** is an anatomically small group of cells located in the medial hypothalamus in the most ventral part of the third ventricle near the entrance of the infundibular recess (Fig. 45a). Arcuate nucleus neurones are responsive to several circulating endocrine hormones, including the gonadal and adrenal steroids, insulin, ghrelin, leptin, the GIT peptide $PYY_{(3-36)}$ and glucose, and the arcuate nucleus may also be an autonomous generator of diurnal rhythms. The arcuate nucleus is part of the central appetite control system through: (i) neuropeptide Y (NPY) and Agouti gene-related peptide (AgRP) neurones, whose stimulation promotes feeding behaviour; and (ii) through pro-opiomelanocortin (POMC) and cocaine and amphetamine-regulated transcript (CART) neurones, whose stimulation inhibits feeding. There is a reciprocal interaction in that activation of NPY/AgRP-expressing neurones inhibits the POMC/CART neurones. Thus, inhibition or destruction of the arcuate nucleus removes an important regulatory control from the lateral hypothalamic centres.

Arcuate NPY/AgRP-expressing neurones and POMC/CART neurones project to the **paraventricular nucleus** (PVN) and to the **lateral hypothalamic area** (LHA) (Fig. 45b), whose destruction, as mentioned above, resulted in loss of feeding behaviour in rats. It is thought that activation of the PVN and LHA by the NPY/AgRP-expressing neurones promotes feeding behaviour through activation of the PVN/LHA centres. Conversely, the POMC/CART-expressing neurones inhibit the PVN/LHA centres. This hypothesis is derived largely from the observation that leptin, the satiety hormone, inhibits the arcuate NPY/AgRP-expressing neurones while activating the arcuate POMC/CART neurones (Fig. 45b).

POMC neurones produce the peptide pro-opiomelanocortin, which is spliced into several other active peptides, including α-MSH (see Chapter 18). α-MSH is believed to be the product responsible, through the agency of the MCR-4 receptor, for the inhibitory action of the POMC system on feeding behaviour. This is far from established, however, since other products of POMC splicing, such as ACTH, γ-LPH and β-MSH may bind the MCR-4 receptor.

Signals from the hypothalamic feeding centres are relayed to the periphery via the brainstem nucleus of the tractus solitarius (NTS), which also receives afferent signals from the GIT via the autonomic nervous system. The GIT sends humoral messages to the central nervous system through several other hormones, including the gastric hormone ghrelin, which activates the NPY/AgRP-expressing neurones while a colon peptide called $PYY_{(3-36)}$, inhibits them.

The LHA produces yet another set of orexigenic peptides called the orexins or hypocretins. (Fig. 45b). Two orexins have been discovered, designated A and B, and appear to mediate food-seeking behaviour, arousal and sleep–wakefulness in several brain areas, through their activation of pathways from the LHA to other brain centres, including the amygdaloid nuclei and the brainstem. The orexin neurones in turn appear to be regulated by humoral cues, including those provided by leptin, glucose, ghrelin, the endocannabinoids and the neurotransmitters norepinephrine and acetylcholine.

In summary, there appears to be a regulatory feedback loop that operates to sustain a balance between energy intake and expenditure (see Fig. 43a). The loop allows the brain to assess the extent of adipose tissue through leptin and govern feeding behaviour accordingly. The situation, particularly in humans, is not as simple as the above would suggest. Leptin production is indeed related to adipose tissue mass; in humans, however, circulating leptin concentrations are not easily related to adiposity. Furthermore, there do not appear to be the short-term changes in circulating leptin that might be expected with intermittent food intake. Also, women generally have higher circulating leptin levels than do men. It is more likely that in humans, leptin forms part of a regulatory system designed to sustain levels of stored energy for the purpose of longer-term survival. Ghrelin may be an endogenous regulator of feeding while peptide PYY may be a medium-term satiety factor.

In humans and possibly other primates, behaviour related to the intake of food has been liberated from the more primitive imperatives of the neuroendocrine loop, analogous to the freedom from imperatives that through hormonal changes allow or forbid female reproductive behaviour. Thus humans can choose to override satiety signals, which may be a factor in the phenomenon of human obesity, although there is some evidence for a genetic predisposition to obesity (see Chapter 46).

(a) Projected obesity in the UK

Note: Figures beyond 1998 were extrapolated on a straight line by the least squares method on the basis of data from 1980

Source: National Audit Office analysis of data from the Health Survey for England

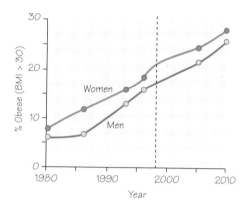

(b) Relationship between body weight, measured by BMI and relative risk

Note: This figure is based on data from a study of female nurses in the United States. Studies for all adults imply a similar relationship between BMI and risk of mortality in men

Source: Manson J.E., Willett M.J. (1995). 'Bodyweight and mortality among women' New England Journal of Medicine

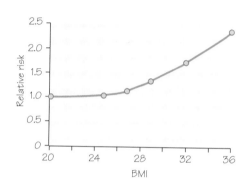

(c) Wild type and Ob/ob mice

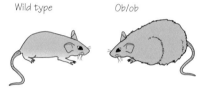

Wild type   Ob/ob

Table 46.1 World Health Organization definition of obesity

Classification	BMI (kg/m²)	Risk of comorbidities
Underweight	<18.5	Low (other clinical problems)
Normal	18.5–24.9	Average
Overweight	25–29.9	Mildly increased
Obese	>30	
Class 1	30–34.9	Moderate
Class 2	35–39.9	Severe
Class 3	>40	Very severe

Table 46.2 Relative risk of different diseases in obese versus nonobese people

Disease	Relative risk		Working days lost
	Women	Men	
Type 2 diabetes	12.7	5.2	5 960 000
Hypertension	4.2	2.6	5 160 000
Heart attack	3.2	1.5	1 230 000
Colon cancer	2.7	3.0	
Angina	1.8	1.8	2 390 000
Gall bladder disease	1.8	1.8	20
Ovarian cancer	1.7		
Osteoarthritis	1.4	1.9	950 000
Stroke	1.3	1.3	440 000
Cancers			970 000

Clinical background

Obesity is a global problem in public health and rates of obesity are increasing throughout the world (Fig. 46a). The World Health Organization has defined obesity as 'abnormal or excessive fat accumulation in adipose tissue to the extent that health is impaired'. Obesity is associated with an increased risk of Type 2 diabetes, hypertension, hyperlipidaemia, cardiovascular disease, sleep apnoea syndrome and respiratory failure, subfertility, arthritis and gallbladder disease. Targets are set using the measurement of Body Mass Index (BMI; weight [kg] / height² [m²]) (Table 46.1).

The relationship between BMI and comorbidities (Fig. 46b) may vary between ethnic groups and certain studies use different cut-off points for that reason. Special charts have been developed to examine obesity rates in children. As central adiposity is associated with a higher risk of metabolic disorders, the waist–hip ratio or straightforward waist measurement has been widely used to identify high-risk groups.

It has been estimated that about 315 million people worldwide fall into the WHO category of obesity. In wealthy societies, all studies report a rate of about 20%, with more women falling into the obesity category but a higher percentage of men found to be overweight (BMI 25–29.9). In the US, around 60% of the population has a BMI >25 kg/m^2 and 27% are obese. Figures from Europe vary between countries and are slightly lower than those seen in the US. In the world's poorer countries there are wide variations, particularly in developing economies. Thus in China the rates of overweight and obesity are increasing, so that around 8–12% of the population are defined as obese. In poor, rural African states obesity rates remain low but recently they have increased dramatically in South Africa; a similar picture related to affluence and urbanization can be seen in Central and South America.

Obesity is the result of complex interactions between genetic, environmental and psychological factors. Our knowledge of some of the genetic factors that play a role in obesity, and the endocrine and metabolic disturbances they induce, has increased dramatically. However, it is clear that the current obesity epidemic has occurred too rapidly for it to be accounted for by changes in the genetic pool. Environmental factors are key to obesity, in particular the reduction in physical activity associated with technological advances and the change to diets rich in saturated fats and sugars.

Introduction

Obesity is becoming widespread in modern human societies, particularly those in which large amounts of carbohydrates and fats are consumed, and is not confined to affluent populations, but also affects those (such as Mexico) in which relatively inexpensive so-called fast foods are heavily marketed. Obesity is strongly linked with several potentially life-threatening cardiovascular and metabolic disorders, including thromboembolic disease and diabetes mellitus (see Chapter 41). A serious manifestation of the growing problem is the appearance of gross obesity and Type 2 diabetes in young children.

Obesity may be defined as excessive amounts of adipose tissue in relation to lean body mass. It may be quantified as the body mass index (BMI; Table 46.1). Waist-to-hip ratio (WHR) is another risk indicator and is the ratio of waist circumference to hip circumference. A ratio of 1 or more indicates risk of heart disease and other obesity-related problems. Generally, large fat deposits on the waist suggest higher risk due to their correlation with insulin resistance than fat on thighs or hips. The cost in health and economic terms is summarized in Table 46.2, compiled by the National Audit Office.

Possible causes of obesity

Social influences. Dietary influences have been referred to above and are doubtless significant causes of obesity. Social factors include the extensive advertising of appetizing foods, drinks and of alcohol and the intrusion of this advertising and of confectionary marketing into schools, a phenomenon now commonplace. Additives such as monosodium glutamate, sucrose, caffeine and a whole array of flavourings render these preparations capable of inducing what is now increasingly referred to, even in the scientific literature, as 'binge eating'. Alcoholic high calorie beverages such as 'alcopops' are aggressively marketed. Furthermore, the stresses of a highly competitive industrial society and of financial insecurity, coupled with changing patterns of personal relationships, may have encouraged the phenomenon of so-called 'comfort eating'.

Evidence for genetic causes of obesity was initially provided by the occurrence of familial obesity, and scientific evidence by the observation of massive obesity in mutant *ob/ob* mice with a recessively inherited disease (Fig. 46c). The mice eat voraciously and develop symptoms of Type 2 diabetes. Apart from their hyperlipidaemia, hyperphagia, hyperglycaemia and insulin resistance, the mice are also hypothermic and infertile. The *ob* gene was cloned and its product expressed and termed **leptin** (Greek *leptos*, which means thin). It is expressed only by fat cells. The role of leptin as an endocrine hormone regulating body weight and energy metabolism through an action in the brain is covered more fully in Chapter 45. The *ob/ob* mice possess two mutant copies of the *ob* gene that do not express leptin, and administration of leptin to these mice reduces food intake, body weight, increases sympathetic nervous activity and lowers circulating insulin levels. The leptin receptor has been found mainly in the brain, although a short splice variant has been found in several tissues in the periphery and in the choroid plexus, where it may mediate the transfer of leptin into the brain.

Another obese mouse mutant, the *db/db* mouse, was found to produce leptin but is unresponsive to it, because it expresses a mutant leptin receptor causing leptin resistance. Leptin receptor mutations have not been found to be causal in human obesity although other target receptors, such as the MCR-4, are under intensive investigation.

Other endocrine hormones which through inappropriate action might contribute to obesity are the adrenal glucocorticoids, growth hormone, insulin, glucagon and thyroxine, all of which play an important part in the regulation of glucose flows and therefore in the integration of fat, carbohydrate and protein metabolism (see Chapter 44).

Autonomic malfunction has also been implicated in obesity in that sympathetic innervation of thermogenic brown adipose tissue is impaired in obese strains of mice, and parasympathetic activity appears to dominate. Further evidence for autonomic involvement was the observation that removal of pancreatic insulin-producing islets and transplantation under the kidney capsule, which removes autonomic influences, reversed the hyperphagia produced by lesions of the ventromedial hypothalamus in rats. In other words, high circulating insulin suppressed the central feeding centres.

47 Obesity: II Cardiovascular and respiratory complications

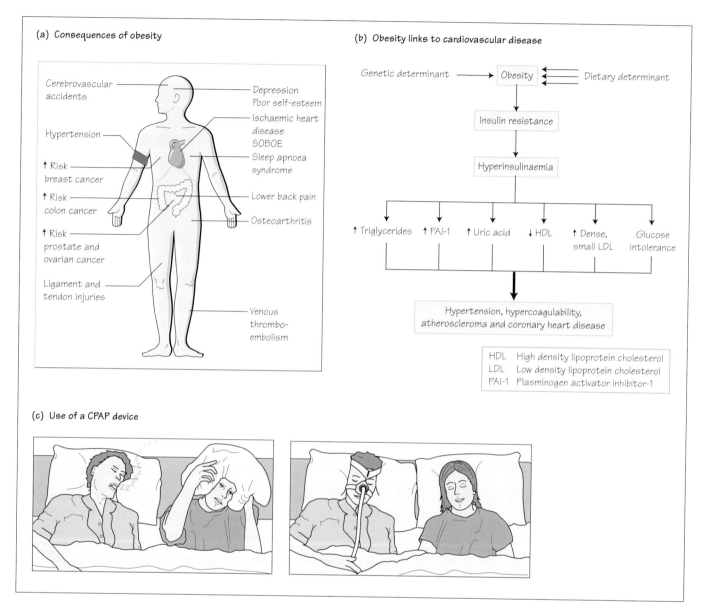

(a) Consequences of obesity

- Cerebrovascular accidents
- Hypertension
- ↑ Risk breast cancer
- ↑ Risk colon cancer
- ↑ Risk prostate and ovarian cancer
- Ligament and tendon injuries
- Depression Poor self-esteem
- Ischaemic heart disease SOBOE
- Sleep apnoea syndrome
- Lower back pain
- Osteoarthritis
- Venous thrombo-embolism

(b) Obesity links to cardiovascular disease

Genetic determinant → Obesity ← Dietary determinant

Obesity → Insulin resistance → Hyperinsulinaemia →

↑ Triglycerides | ↑ PAI-1 | ↑ Uric acid | ↓ HDL | ↑ Dense, small LDL | Glucose intolerance

→ Hypertension, hypercoagulability, atheroscleroma and coronary heart disease

HDL   High density lipoprotein cholesterol
LDL   Low density lipoprotein cholesterol
PAI-1 Plasminogen activator inhibitor-1

(c) Use of a CPAP device

Clinical background

Obesity is associated with a number of complications and comorbidities. Cardiovascular disease is the major cause of death in obese patients and there is a direct link between the degree of obesity and the degree of hypertension. Other risk factors for coronary heart disease, such as smoking and hyperlipidaemia, should be addressed. There is also a higher risk of thromboembolism and stroke in the obese population. Other complications include osteoarthritis, back pain, ligament and tendon injury, gallstones and an increased risk of certain cancers, in particular those of the colon, rectum, breast, endometrium and prostate (Fig. 47a). Sleep apnoea syndrome is more common in the obese, particularly men.

Cardiovascular complications of obesity

Obesity not only relates to but also predicts coronary atherosclerosis in both men and women, even with minimal increases in BMI (Fig. 47b). Disordered lipid metabolism occurs partly through decreased levels of the enzyme lipoprotein lipase, an insulin-sensitive enzyme that breaks down fat. This results in elevated serum triglycerides and reduced HDL cholesterol. Hyperglycaemia results in the glycation of more LDL, which increases the affinity of LDL for the modified LDL receptors on macrophages. This in turn promotes endothelial cell cytotoxicity, foam cell production and smooth muscle proliferation. Plasminogen activator inhibitor (PAI-1) is raised (Fig. 47b), and this prothrombic state is a further risk factor for coronary artery disease. Elevated circulating levels of C-reactive protein, a systemic marker of inflammation, also occur as increased visceral fat appears to enhance the inflammatory pathway response that involves phospholipase A2, intracellular adhesion molecule and C-reactive protein.

Congestive cardiac failure. Left ventricular hypertrophy is a common feature of obesity. In the absence of hypertension, increases in cardiac output and stroke volume with diastolic dysfunction and have been related to sudden death in obese patients. Changes in the right heart are also seen in obese patients. These changes may occur as a consequence of sleep apnoea and the obesity hypoventilation syndrome, and result in right ventricular hypertrophy and pulmonary hypertension, and eventual failure. Right ventricular dysfunction may also occur as a result of left ventricular dysfunction, with subsequent biventricular failure.

Hypertension is often a consequence of obesity, particularly in patients who have also developed hyperinsulinaemia and hypertriglyceridaemia. These patients will be predisposed to myocardial infarction, stroke and renal failure. Obesity-related hypertension is of complex aetiology. Free fatty acids, leptin and insulin may all be raised in the patient's blood and may act together to activate the renin–angiotensin system and promote sympathetic activity with consequent vasoconstriction and sodium retention.

It has been found, using animal models of obesity, that obesity causes inflammatory changes in small blood vessel walls with adverse consequences for perfusion of vascular beds.

Respiratory complications of obesity

Sleep apnoea describes the cessation of breathing during sleep. This syndrome is characterized by snoring and apnoeic episodes culminating in sudden waking associated with a rise in arterial $P_a CO_2$. Patients may experience many apnoeic episodes in a single night, resulting in severe sleep disturbance and daytime somnolence. Fat deposition in the neck may externally compress the upper airways and infiltration of adipose tissue into muscle may decrease upper airway size, render the pharynx more susceptible to collapse and decrease chest wall compliance. Furthermore, abdominal fat may impede diaphragmatic movement, especially in the supine position. In obesity hypoventilation syndrome, there may also be a reduced central respiratory drive.

Detailed sleep studies should be performed as, untreated, sleep apnoea syndrome may lead to the development of pulmonary hypertension and right heart failure. Machines exerting continuous positive airway pressure (CPAP; Fig. 47c) are available which effectively 'splint' the upper airways preventing their collapse. These provide relief for sufferers of sleep apnoea, and also for their partners.

48 Obesity: III Insulin resistance and endocrine complications

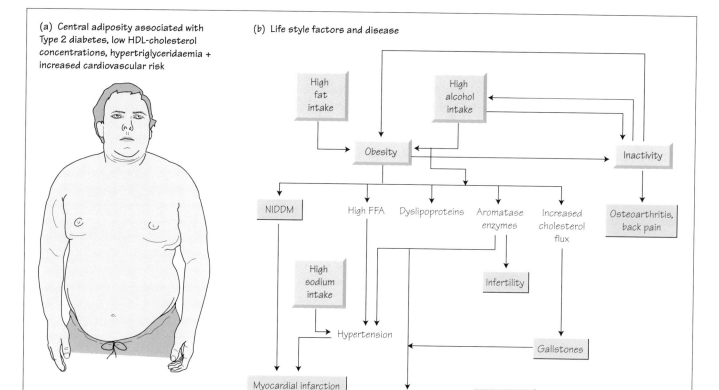

(a) Central adiposity associated with Type 2 diabetes, low HDL-cholesterol concentrations, hypertriglyceridaemia + increased cardiovascular risk

(b) Life style factors and disease

Table 48.1 Metabolic consequences of obesity

Type 2 diabetes
Raised serum triglycerides
Low high-density lipoprotein (HDL) cholesterol
Hyperinsulinaemia and insulin resistance
Raised plasma fibrinogen levels

Red boxes – important diseases
Green boxes – lifestyle factors which predispose to the diseases
NIDDM   Non-insulin dependent diabetes mellitus
FFA   Free fatty acid

Clinical background

Metabolic syndrome

Obesity is associated with a number of metabolic consequences characterized by insulin resistance and hyperlipidaemia. These in turn contribute to the increased risk of cardiovascular disease and diabetes (Fig. 48a and Table 48.1). Metabolic syndrome is the term given to a range of metabolic disturbances occurring in the same patient, all of which should be addressed and modified. Patients with metabolic syndrome have insulin resistance, which precedes the onset of hypertension and Type 2 DM and is thought to represent the primary pathological disturbance. Metabolic syndrome thus describes insulin resistance, hyperinsulinaemia, hypertension, hypertriglyceridaemia, low HDL-cholesterol and obesity. Patients with metabolic syndrome are at a high risk of macrovascular disease and treatment should be aimed at improving insulin sensitivity by diet and exercise and aggressive treatment of hyperlipidaemia.

Polycystic ovary syndrome and insulin resistance

Obesity is found in around 50% of women with polycystic ovary syndrome (PCOS; see Chapter 26). Furthermore, lean women with PCOS demonstrate lesser degrees of hyperinsulinaemia and insulin resistance, which play a role in the pathogenesis of PCOS independently of obesity as insulin stimulates ovarian androgen production. The metabolic consequences of obesity and hyperinsulinaemia are seen in women with PCOS who have a high risk of developing impaired glucose tolerance and Type 2 diabetes. Clinical evidence of hyperinsulinaemia may be seen as acanthosis nigricans, a brown velvety pigmentation usually seen at the base of the neck and in the axillae in obese women with PCOS.

Other endocrine causes and implications of obesity

Other endocrine causes and implications of obesity include Cushing's syndrome (see Chapter 17) and hypothyroidism (see Chapter 14). Cushing's syndrome largely reflects the symptoms produced by excess cortisol secretion in to the circulation, although the obesity produced is due to redistribution of fat to the face, neck and abdominal region. There is also significant fluid retention with attendant cardiovascular problems due to the mineralocorticoid action of cortisol when present in the blood in high concentrations. Hypothyroidism may be associated with weight gain. Obesity distorts results from tests of hypothalamo–pituitary function. Provocative tests are often impaired. For example obesity blunts the response of GH release to a challenge of GHRH. The cortisol response to CRH is also impaired in obese patients, and these abnormal responses disappear with a reduction in weight.

Treatment of obesity

Obesity is a chronic disorder associated with significant morbidity, impaired quality of life and increased mortality rates. Treatment of obesity is difficult, not only due to the need for obese individuals to make significant lifestyle changes (Fig. 48b), but also due to prejudices held by society and doctors towards the condition and its management. The principle of treating obesity is simple – to produce a negative energy balance that utilizes body stores and is maintained in the long term. The practice is more complex, requiring education about diet and activity levels and, where deemed necessary, the introduction of pharmacological agents in addition to lifestyle modification.

Orlistat, inhibits pancreatic lipase thus reducing gastrointestinal fat absorption has been shown to be effective and is licensed for use in the UK. Research into a number of other agents continues, such as leptin and neuropeptide Y antagonists. Surgical therapy such as gastric banding to reduce gastric size remains an option for patients with morbid obesity who have failed dietary and medical interventions and is the most effective treatment for individuals with a BMI $>40 \, kg \, m^2$

49 Calcium: I Parathyroid hormone

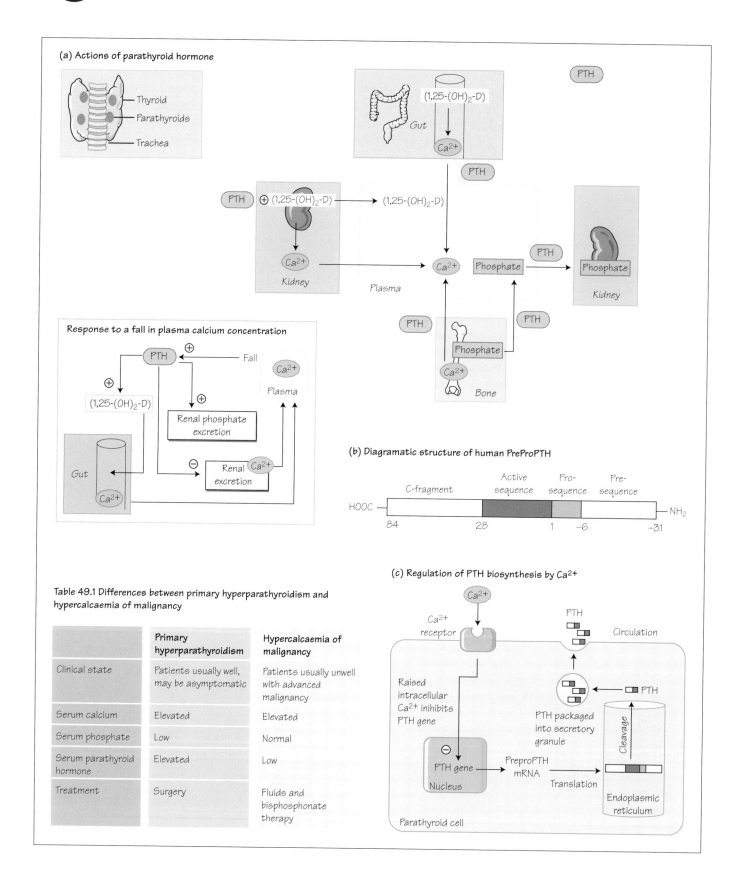

(a) Actions of parathyroid hormone

Response to a fall in plasma calcium concentration

(b) Diagramatic structure of human PreProPTH

(c) Regulation of PTH biosynthesis by Ca^{2+}

Table 49.1 Differences between primary hyperparathyroidism and hypercalcaemia of malignancy

	Primary hyperparathyroidism	Hypercalcaemia of malignancy
Clinical state	Patients usually well, may be asymptomatic	Patients usually unwell with advanced malignancy
Serum calcium	Elevated	Elevated
Serum phosphate	Low	Normal
Serum parathyroid hormone	Elevated	Low
Treatment	Surgery	Fluids and bisphosphonate therapy

Clinical scenario

A 55-year-old woman, Mrs CB, had a routine blood test at her general practitioners and was found to have a serum calcium level of 2.88 mmol/L. She was referred to the local endocrine clinic. She was completely asymptomatic, having none of the classical symptoms associated with hypercalcaemia such as bone pain, abdominal pains, renal colic, thirst, polyuria or tiredness. Further investigations confirmed a high serum calcium in association with a low serum phosphate, normal Vitamin D concentrations, a raised 24-hour urine calcium excretion and an elevated serum parathyroid hormone concentration. Sestamibi radioisotope scanning revealed a single abnormality in the upper right parathyroid gland and subsequent surgery confirmed the presence of a single parathyroid adenoma.

Role of calcium

Calcium is essential for: bone growth, blood clotting, maintenance of the transmembrane potential, cell replication, stimulus–contraction and stimulus–secretion coupling, and the second messenger process.

Circulating and extracellular calcium, in adult humans, is kept at 2.2–2.6 mmol/L. This equilibrium is achieved mainly in the kidney and the digestive tract, and by an exchange between bone and extracellular fluid. About half the circulating ion is free and the rest is bound to plasma albumin. Circulating calcium equilibrium is upset by protein abnormalities, acid–base disturbances, and by changes in the concentrations of plasma albumin. Bone provides the largest pool of calcium, a smaller pool is provided by the soft tissues and an even smaller pool by the extracellular fluid. Children are in a positive calcium balance, and over the first 18 years postnatally they will retain about 1 kg of calcium.

Regulation of calcium metabolism

This is principally through three hormones: parathyroid hormone (PTH), from the parathyroid gland (Fig. 49a), which raises circulating calcium concentrations; calcitonin from the parafollicular cells of the thyroid, which lowers calcium; and 1,25-dihydroxy-vitamin D_3, a metabolite of vitamin D, which increases circulating calcium ions.

The parathyroid glands are present in all terrestrial vertebrates. In humans, there are four parathyroid glands embedded one at each pole of the thyroid gland and consisting of adipocytes and chief cells, which synthesize the hormone. There are other cells, called oxyphil cells, which increase in number after puberty, and whose function is unknown. **Parathyroid hormone** is also called parathormone and is abbreviated to PTH.

Synthesis and secretion of PTH

The PTH gene is localized to the short arm of chromosome 11. Mature PTH is a polypeptide of 84 amino acids, cleaved from a pro-PTH of 90 amino acids, which in turn is cleaved from a prepro-PTH of 115 amino acids (Fig. 49b). Cleavage of pro-PTH to PTH occurs about 15 minutes after arrival at the Golgi apparatus of pro-PTH, which is packaged in vesicles and released by exocytosis.

Secretion is controlled by plasma calcium such that there is an inverse relationship between plasma calcium and PTH (Fig. 49c). The parathyroid chief cells have recognition sites for calcium and the second messenger appears to be cAMP. PTH is cleaved in the circulation, the liver and the kidney, and one of the circulating fragments (1–34) retains biological activity.

Physiological actions of PTH

Bone. PTH acts on bone to liberate calcium, orthophosphate, magnesium, citrate, hydroxyproline and osteocalcin, which forms 1–28% of all bone protein and has a high affinity for calcium. PTH therefore has a resorptive effect on bone, which is probably directly on the osteoblasts, which then stimulate osteoclast activity. Osteoblasts synthesize collagen, on which calcium phosphate precipitates as hydroxyapatite crystals. Bone is demineralized by the osteoclast cells, which release hyaluronic acid and acid phosphatase, which solubilize calcium phosphate.

Gastrointestinal tract. PTH stimulates the uptake of calcium from the GIT by an indirect action on vitamin D metabolism.

Kidney. PTH enhances the urinary excretion of phosphate through a direct action on the proximal tubules of the kidney (Fig. 49a). This stimulates calcium resorption of bone because it promotes calcium ionization through the reduction in the $[Ca^{2+}] \times [PO_4^{3-}]$ solubility product. In addition, PTH inhibits bicarbonate reabsorption, stimulating a metabolic acidosis which favours calcium ionization, resorption of calcium from bone, and dissociation of calcium from plasma protein binding sites.

Pathophysiology of PTH

Hypercalcaemia is a common endocrine disorder. The vast majority (97%) are either due to primary hyperparathyroidism or the hypercalcaemia associated with malignancy (Table 49.1). Rarely, hypercalcaemia is caused by sarcoidosis, untreated renal failure, thyrotoxicosis, ingestion of excess milk, alkali or vitamin D or by prolonged immobilization. The symptoms of hypercalcaemia include polyuria, polydipsia, bone pain, abdominal pain due to renal stones and depression. There may be radiological evidence of bone resorption, particularly in the terminal phalanges.

Hyperparathyroidism. Most patients with primary hyperparathyroidism are found to have a benign parathyroid adenoma. More rarely, four gland parathyroid hyperplasia or (very rarely) a parathyroid carcinoma may be found. In patients with a single parathyroid adenoma, occasionally conservative management with monitoring of the calcium is appropriate, particularly in the elderly. However, in general, surgical removal is advised to prevent the onset of bone disease in the long term.

Secondary hyperparathyroidism occurs after prolonged hypocalcaemia, usually seen in chronic renal failure.

Hypoparathyroidism or PTH deficiency leads to hypocalcaemia. Primary hypoparathyroidism is a rare condition of autoimmune origin; more commonly hypoparathyroidism occurs following thyroid surgery and inadvertent damage to the parathyroid glands.

(a) Calcitonin synthesis

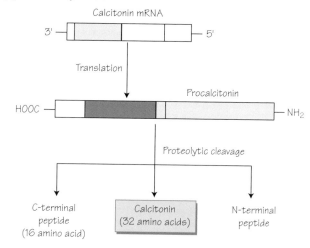

Calcitonin mRNA

3' — 5'

↓ Translation

HOOC — Procalcitonin — NH₂

↓ Proteolytic cleavage

C-terminal peptide (16 amino acid) — Calcitonin (32 amino acids) — N-terminal peptide

(b) Role of calcitonin

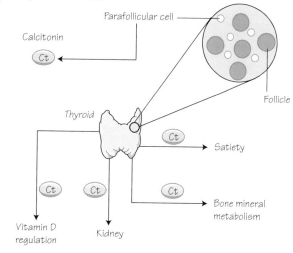

Parafollicular cell

Calcitonin
Ct

Thyroid

Follicle

Ct → Satiety

Ct   Ct   Ct → Bone mineral metabolism

Vitamin D regulation   Kidney

Table 50.1 Multiple Endocrine Neoplasia Syndromes

Multiple Endocrine Neoplasia (MEN) describes the occurrence of tumours in two or more endocrine organs in the same patient. There are two main types depending on the glands involved, MEN 1 (associated with mutations in chromosome 11q13) and MEN 2, the latter being divided into three subgroups, MEN 2a and 2b and Medullary Thyroid Cancer (MTC) only. The gene causing the MEN 2 syndromes is mapped to chromosome 10cen-10q11. MEN syndromes may be familial or sporadic although care should be taken in describing disease as sporadic – the family member with the disease may have died before it was diagnosed

Clinical features

MEN 1 Tumours of the parathyroids, pancreas and pituitary, rarely adrenal cortex, carcinomas and lipomas

MEN 2a MTC, phaeochromocytomas, parathyroid hyperplasia/tumours

MEN 2b As MEN 2a with additional associated abnormalities such as mucosal neuromas, Marfanoid features

Clinical background

Medullary thyroid cancer (MTC) is a rare malignancy arising from the parafollicular thyroid C cells that secrete calcitonin. It usually presents as a lump in the thyroid gland or as lymph node metastases in the neck. Diagnosis is made by a biopsy and the treatment is surgical, possibly with adjunctive chemotherapy. MTC may be sporadic or familial and in both types may be associated with phaeochromocytoma or other features of the Multiple Endocrine Neoplasia Type 2 (MEN 2) syndrome (Table 50.1). It is important to distinguish the truly sporadic cases from the first presentation of familial disease as screening can allow early detection and treatment in family members.

Calcitonin

Calcitonin is a hypocalcaemic polypeptide hormone. In mammals, it is synthesized and secreted in parafollicular (C) cells in the thyroid gland. C cells have been found in much lower density in the parathyroid glands and in the thymus. In fish and birds, calcitonin is synthesized within a specific organ, the ultimobranchial body. The ultimobranchial bodies do develop in mammals during fetal life, but eventually disappear. It is thought that the C cells evolved before the parathyroids, to help sea-dwelling animals to cope with the relatively high concentrations of calcium in sea water.

Biosynthesis and secretion. The calcitonin gene occurs on the short arm of chromosome 11. Calcitonin (CT) is synthesized in C (clear) cells from a larger 136 amino acid precursor, called calcitonin precursor, from which CT is cleaved, together with two other peptides of unknown function (Fig. 50a). The gene which encodes CT has been characterized, and is expressed not only in the C cells of the thyroid but also in the brain. In neural tissue, however, the gene expresses not CT but another peptide, the calcitonin gene-related peptide (CGRP). This is therefore an example of tissue-determining expression of a common gene.

At normal plasma calcium levels, CT release is low but a rise in calcium causes a rapid (threefold) rise in CT concentrations.

Even if a small amount of calcium, which is insufficient to raise plasma concentrations of the ion in plasma, reaches the gastrointestinal tract (GIT), CT is released. It is therefore thought that other GIT factors, for example gastrin and/or cholecystokinin (CCK), may trigger CT secretion. The sensitivity of the CT-release mechanism is sexually differentiated, being greater in males, and the responsiveness of the CT release mechanism declines with ageing. The half-life of CT in plasma is less than 15 minutes, and it may be degraded and excreted principally by the kidney.

Physiological actions of calcitonin (Fig. 50b). In humans, calcitonin is not as important as is PTH in the regulation of calcium metabolism. The two main target organs for CT are **bone** and **kidney**. In bone, CT is a potent inhibitor of resorption, both *in vivo* and *in vitro*, although CT has no effects on bone formation. There is an inhibition of calcium resorption by the osteoclasts within 20 minutes of administration of a dose of CT. CT may be particularly important during periods of threatened increased calcium loss, such as occurs during pregnancy and lactation.

In the kidney, CT is concentrated in the renal cortex. Membranes of the tubule cells possess specific CT receptors, and the second messenger may be adenylate cyclase, although administration of CT does not appear to alter cellular levels of cAMP. In the kidney, CT increases the excretion of calcium, sodium and potassium and reduces excretion of magnesium.

CT may be important in the regulation of postprandial feeding, to prevent food-induced hypercalcaemia. CT may also be a satiety hormone. In humans, injection of CT is followed by a significant fall in body weight within 36 hours, and CT inhibits feeding behaviour in rhesus monkeys and rats. The hormone is particularly potent when administered directly to the brain, suggesting that it may have a central role.

CT affects **vitamin D** metabolism by lowering plasma calcium, resulting in the release of PTH, which in turn promotes the production and secretion of vitamin D metabolites in the kidney.

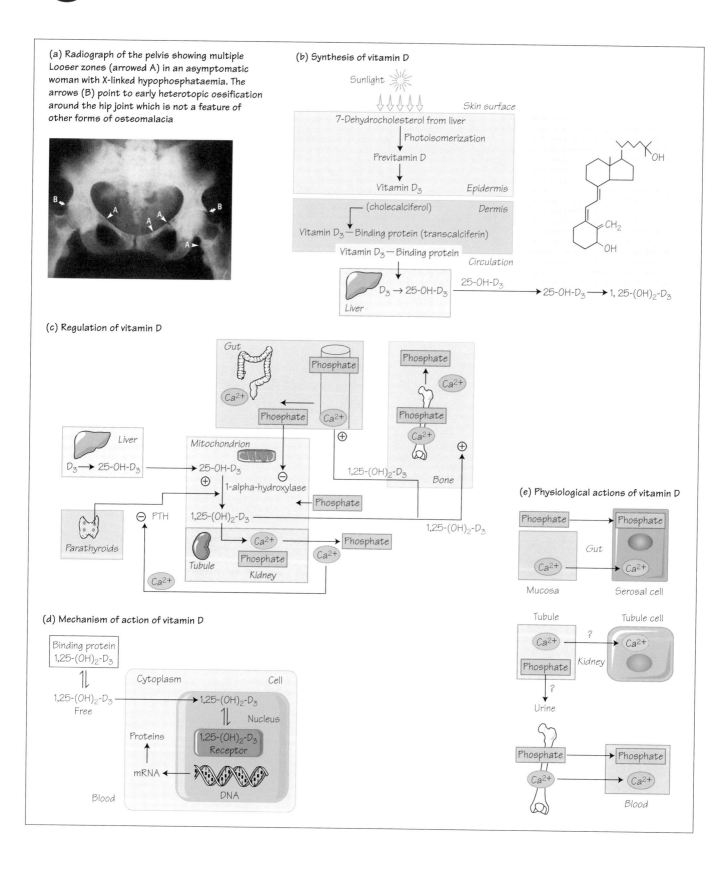

(a) Radiograph of the pelvis showing multiple Looser zones (arrowed A) in an asymptomatic woman with X-linked hypophosphataemia. The arrows (B) point to early heterotopic ossification around the hip joint which is not a feature of other forms of osteomalacia

(b) Synthesis of vitamin D

(c) Regulation of vitamin D

(d) Mechanism of action of vitamin D

(e) Physiological actions of vitamin D

Clinical scenario

Mrs BK, a 55-year-old lady of Bangladeshi origin, presented to her GP complaining of various non-specific symptoms including generalized aches and pains and muscle weakness when walking, particularly going upstairs. Investigations showed her to have a serum calcium level of 2.02 mmol/L in association with a raised alkaline phosphatase of 358 U/L and an elevated PTH concentration. Serum vitamin D concentrations were measured and found to be below the seasonal normal range. Her symptoms resolved with calcium and vitamin D supplementation.

Vitamin D deficiency is common, particularly in patients of Asian background and the elderly living alone on poor diets. In northern European populations there is a marked seasonal variation in normal serum concentrations related to varying daylight lengths. Low vitamin D levels cause hypocalcaemia, compensated for by the development of secondary hyperparathyroidism which maintains the serum calcium at low normal or mildly suppressed levels. Untreated, vitamin D deficiency can lead to the development of rickets in children or osteomalacia in adults (Fig. 51a), both associated with characteristic bone abnormalities. Recently an increase in vitamin D deficiency has been noted in children from more affluent European backgrounds with limited sun exposure due to overzealous sun protection.

Vitamin D

Vitamins are not generally considered to be hormones, but organic dietary factors essential for healthy life. The term 'vitamin' is perhaps a misnomer therefore for the substances called vitamin D. The term 'vitamin D' refers to two steroid-like chemicals, namely **ergocalciferol** and **cholecalciferol**. Osteomalacia is the softening of bones in adults who suffer from a deficiency of vitamin D in the diet, or of sunlight, or both.

Synthesis of vitamin D

The active form of vitamin D is 1-alpha, 25-dihydroxyvitamin D_3 (1,25-$(OH)_2$-D_3). Ultraviolet irradiation in sunlight photoisomerizes a cholesterol precursor, 7-dehydrocholesterol, which converts it to previtamin D, which then undergoes a thermal isomerization to cholecalciferol (vitamin D_3; Fig. 51b). Cholecalciferol binds in the dermis to a binding protein, which transports it in the plasma, and it is converted in the liver to 25-hydroxyvitamin D_3 (25-OH-D_3). This metabolite circulates, and in the kidney it is converted into the active metabolite 1,25-$(OH)_2$-D_3.

Regulation of metabolism

The regulation of vitamin D_3 metabolism is linked to parathyroid hormone (PTH; Fig. 51c). PTH secretion from the parathyroid glands is stimulated by hypocalcaemia. PTH stimulates the kidney cortex mitochondrial enzyme 1-alpha-hydroxylase, which is also stimulated by low concentrations of phosphate. The 1,25-$(OH)_2$-D_3 thus formed enters the circulation and promotes calcium resorption from bone. Calcium absorption from the gastrointestinal tract (GIT) stimulates the reabsorption of calcium from the kidney and the excretion of phosphate. The hypercalcaemia created inhibits further production of PTH, which in turn limits the synthesis of 1,25-$(OH)_2$-D_3. The active metabolite is inactivated by conversion to 24,25-$(OH)_2$-D_3. 1,25-$(OH)_2$-D_3 may also feed back to the parathyroid glands to inhibit the release of PTH. The glands do possess receptors for 1,25-$(OH)_2$-D_3.

Mechanism of action

The 1,25-$(OH)_2$-D_3 receptor belongs to a superfamily of nuclear hormone receptors, which bind to their ligand and alter transcription (see Chapter 4). The hormone travels in the bloodstream in equilibrium between bound and free forms. The latter form is freely able to enter cells, due to its lipophilic nature. The plasma 1,25-$(OH)_2$-D_3-binding protein (DBP) recognizes the hormone specifically. 1,25-$(OH)_2$-D_3 binds to the nuclear receptor; the complex binds to specific hormone response elements on the target gene upstream of transcriptional activation sites, and new mRNA and protein synthesis result (Fig. 51d). New proteins synthesized include osteocalcin, an important bone protein whose synthesis is suppressed by glucocorticoids. In the GIT, a calcium-binding transport protein (CaBP) is synthesized in response to the hormone–receptor activation of the genome.

Physiological actions of vitamin D

Bone. Vitamin D stimulates resorption of calcium from bone as part of its function to maintain adequate circulating concentrations of the ion (Fig. 51e). It also stimulates osteocalcin synthesis.

Gastrointestinal tract. 1,25-$(OH)_2$-D_3 stimulates calcium and phosphate absorption from the gut through an active transport process. The hormone promotes the synthesis of calcium transport by enhancing synthesis of the cytosolic calcium-binding protein CaBP, which transports calcium from the mucosal to the serosal cells of the gut.

Kidney. 1,25-$(OH)_2$-D_3 may stimulate reabsorption of calcium into the tubule cells while promoting the excretion of phosphate. The tubule cells do possess receptors for vitamin D and CaBP.

Muscle. Muscle cells have vitamin D receptors, and the hormone may mediate muscle contraction through effects on the calcium fluxes, and on consequent adenosine triphosphate (ATP) synthesis.

Pregnancy. During pregnancy, there is increased calcium absorption from the GIT, and elevated circulating concentrations of 1,25-$(OH)_2$-D_3, DBP, calcitonin and PTH. During the last 6 months prior to birth, calcium and phosphorus accumulate in the fetus. The placenta synthesizes 1,25-$(OH)_2$-D_3, as does the fetal kidney and bone. Nevertheless, the fetus still requires maternal vitamin D.

Other roles. Vitamin D may be involved in the maturation and proliferation of cells of the immune system, for example of the haematopoietic stem cells, and in the function of mature B and T cells.

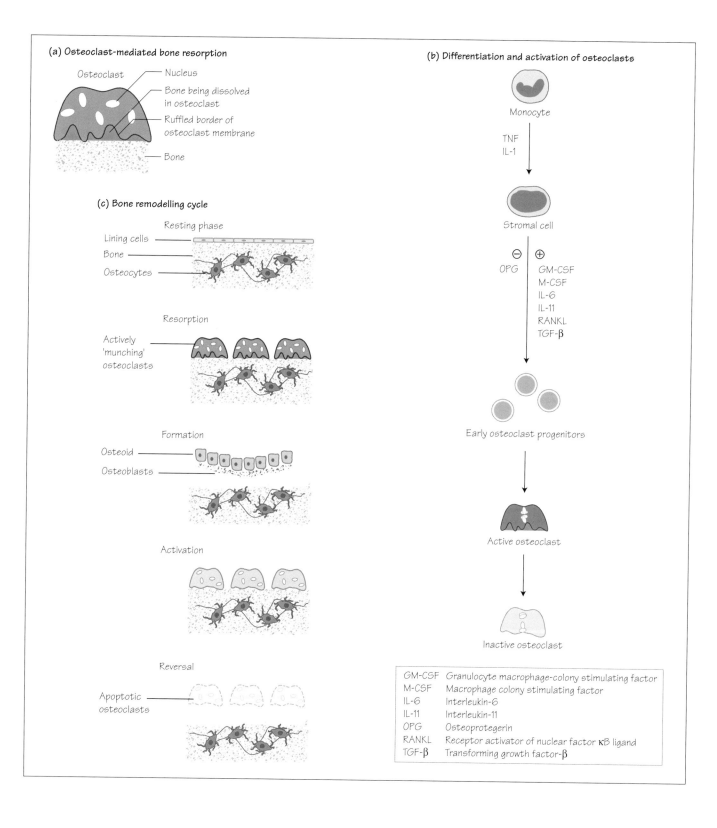

(a) Osteoclast-mediated bone resorption

Osteoclast
Nucleus
Bone being dissolved in osteoclast
Ruffled border of osteoclast membrane
Bone

(c) Bone remodelling cycle

Resting phase

Lining cells
Bone
Osteocytes

Resorption

Actively 'munching' osteoclasts

Formation

Osteoid
Osteoblasts

Activation

Reversal

Apoptotic osteoclasts

(b) Differentiation and activation of osteoclasts

Monocyte

TNF
IL-1

Stromal cell

⊖ ⊕
OPG | GM-CSF
M-CSF
IL-6
IL-11
RANKL
TGF-β

Early osteoclast progenitors

Active osteoclast

Inactive osteoclast

GM-CSF	Granulocyte macrophage-colony stimulating factor
M-CSF	Macrophage colony stimulating factor
IL-6	Interleukin-6
IL-11	Interleukin-11
OPG	Osteoprotegerin
RANKL	Receptor activator of nuclear factor κB ligand
TGF-β	Transforming growth factor-β

Introduction

The nature of bone. Bone is an essential rigid support for the body, a means of effecting locomotion and a reservoir of ions such as calcium, phosphate, magnesium and sodium. Bone is two-thirds mineral and the rest is mainly type 1 collagen and water. Bone mineral is present mainly as crystalline hydroxyapatite and the rest as amorphous calcium phosphate, which occurs in higher amounts in actively forming, young bone.

Bone needs to be not only rigid and strong but also light enough to allow muscle contractions. These properties are conferred by the structure of bone, which in the case of cortical tubular bones consists mainly of densely packed layers of mineralized collagen, and, in the case of the axial skeleton, of spongier trabecular or cancellous bone. Defective cortical bone results in long bone fracture, while defective trabecular bone results in vertebral fractures.

Cellular structure of bone

Bone matrix is laid down in concentric layers called lamellae. The unit of structure in compact bone is the osteon. In each osteon, lamellae are arranged around the central Haversian canal; the canal houses blood vessels and nerves. The osteocytes are located in the lacunae, which are connected by branching tubules called canaliculi. The canaliculi radiate out from the lacunae to form an extensive network, connecting bone cells to each other and to the blood supply.

Cell types in bone

The three main cell types in bone are the osteoblast, osteocyte and osteoclast. The **osteoblast** is the main bone-producing cell. It originates in the bone marrow and when mature possesses receptors for, amongst other hormones, vitamin D and parathyroid hormone (PTH). The differentiated, mature osteoblast migrates to the surface of bone and lays down bone matrix in lamellae and induces mineralization. It expresses alkaline phosphatase and a number of matrix proteins, including osteocalcin and type 1 collagen. **Osteocytes** are osteoblasts entrapped in cortical bone during remodelling; these develop processes which communicate with other osteocytes and with capillaries, thus ensuring a supply of nutrients.

Osteoclasts are large, multinucleated cells whose function is the resorption of bone (Fig. 52a). They originate from haematopoietic mononuclear precursors of the monocyte/macrophage lineage under the influence of interleukin-1 (IL-1) and tumour necrosis factor (TNF) and differentiate under the influence of a number of factors including: macrophage colony-stimulating factor (M-CSF, also called CSF-1); GM-CSF (granulocyte macrophage colony stimulating factor); TGF-b (transforming growth factor-b); IL-6 and IL-11; vitamin D and PTH (Fig. 52b). There is evidence that megakaryocyte cells express the receptor activator of NF-kB ligand (RANKL), a member of the TNF ligand family, which is essential for the differentiation

process. RANKL attaches to RANK, a receptor on the cell surface of osteoclasts and osteoclast precursors, to stimulate proliferation and differentiation of cells to form the osteoclast. Osteoprotegerin (OPG) is a soluble decoy receptor produced by osteoblasts, marrow stromal cells and other cells. It profoundly modifies the effects of RANKL by inhibiting RANKL/RANK interaction. Osteoclasts do not appear to have receptors for vitamin D or PTH. Osteoclasts resorb bone by attaching themselves to bone matrix, breaking it down with catheptic proteases and dissolving it in acid (Fig. 52a). After the osteoclast has attached itself to bone, it seals off the underlying portion from the rest of the bone and develops an invaginated border called the 'ruffled border', which acts as a large lysosome, dissolving the surrounded portion of bone. Resorption can be reduced by reducing the rate of osteoclast formation or by reducing osteoclast activity.

Bone remodelling

Bone remodelling is the cycle of bone resorption and new bone deposition. The cycle depends on systemic hormone action for an adequate supply of calcium phosphate and on local hormone action for communication between osteoblasts and osteoclasts. The balance between mineral supply to the bone and bone resorption under the influence of PTH is normally balanced by chemical signal coupling, which at present is poorly understood. Bone remodelling is a continuous process, so that as bone is being resorbed, new bone (osteoid) is being laid down by osteoblasts (Fig. 52c). In cortical bone, remodelling occurs from within and four phases can be identified: there is a resting phase, while osteoclasts become activated; during the resorption phase, groups of osteoclasts cut tunnels through the bone, followed by trailing osteoblasts; during the reversal phase, the osteoclasts undergo apoptosis; and during the formation phase the osteoblasts lay down new bone.

In cortical bone, osteoblasts lay down cylinders of new bone, progressively narrowing the tunnel, which ultimately becomes the Haversian canal. In trabecular bone, remodelling takes place at the surface, when osteoclasts burrow a pit which is then filled in by osteoblasts.

For both types of bone, the remodelling cycle takes about 200 days. The system is integrated by local chemical signals which have not yet been fully identified but may involve the integrins, the RANKL system and calcitonin, PTH and the interleukins. PTH promotes resorption in order to rectify hypocalcaemia and this triggers osteoblast action. Osteoblasts have receptors for PTH and this may be part of the system that activates the osteoblast. Other hormones undoubtedly influence the system. Estrogens, for example, directly inhibit osteoclastogenensis and have other regulatory effects on osteoblasts and bone marrow stromal cells. Estrogens reveal their profound influence through the osteoporosis which may follow their absence after menopause (see Chapter 54).

53 Metabolic bone disease: I Paget's disease

(a) Facial appearance in Paget's disease showing frontal bossing of skull

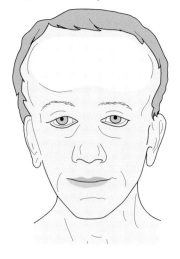

(c) Isotope bone scan showing diffuse uptake in Paget's disease

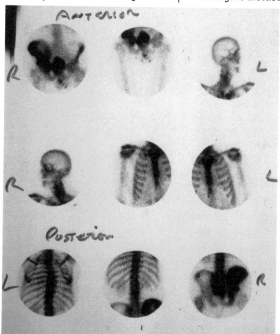

(b) X-ray to show extensive Paget's in the right hemipelvis

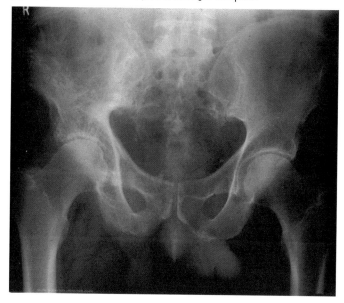

Clinical background

Paget's disease (*osteitis deformans*) is a chronic bone disorder resulting in bone pain and deformity. It affects up to 10% of the elderly, more commonly men, although it may be asymptomatic and discovered on a routine blood test or X-ray. Most commonly patients present with bone pain or deformity – these are characteristic of the disorder and include bowing of the long bones, skull enlargement with frontal bossing and, less commonly, pathological fractures (Fig. 53a, b and c).

Paget's disease is characterized by abnormal bone remodelling. Often the disease is picked up by the finding of a high alkaline phosphatase on biochemical screening. Calcium and PTH concentrations are normal but measurements of markers of bone turnover, such as serum bone-specific alkaline phosphatase (BAP) and osteocalcin indicating bone formation and urinary deoxypyridinoline and N-terminal telopeptide indicating bone resorption, may be helpful.

Patients with Paget's disease are treated with analgesics and bisphosphonates. The latter will reduce bone turnover and improve symptoms. There is an increased risk of malignant change in pagetic bones and any change in symptoms, such as the development of acute pain, heat or fracture in a patient with long-standing disease should be investigated immediately.

Paget's disease of bone

Aetiology and pathology. Paget's disease is a relatively rare disorder of bone remodelling that involves greatly accelerated rates of bone turnover, abnormal bone architecture and may lead to gross bone deformity. It is not strictly a metabolic disorder since the disease is focal to bone. The aetiology is poorly understood but may involve a chronic viral infection since inclusion bodies resembling paramyxovirus have been found in pagetic osteoclasts. The disease may be familial and several genetic associations have been identified. Paget's disease is characterized by features of high metabolic bone activity, including excessive cellularity and vascularity. The osteoclasts, large multinucleate cells which are normally present only when bone is being resorbed, may be huge and highly multinucleate in Paget's disease, when bone is being haphazardly remodelled. The resultant bone, as with other conditions involving high bone turnover, may be so-called woven bone, which lacks the normal lamellar structure. The spine, sacrum and femur are the most frequency affected bones, followed by the skull and pelvis.

Recent advances in the identification of hormones and cytokines involved in the modulation of osteoclastogenesis may throw light on the aetiology of Paget's disease.

Complications of Paget's disease reflect the implications of bone deformity on associated soft tissues, and may be neoplastic, rheumatological, neurological and, rarely, cardiac. The spinal cord and brain are at risk of compression, especially the brain stem and cranial nerves, and deafness often results through effects on the skull. Spinal stenosis (narrowing) may occur in vertebral Paget's disease, and peripheral nerve entrapment may cause, for example, carpal tunnel syndrome. Osteoarthritis is a common complication of Paget's disease and bone sarcoma may develop. Very occasionally, patients may suffer high-output congestive heart failure because of the abnormally high blood flow to bone.

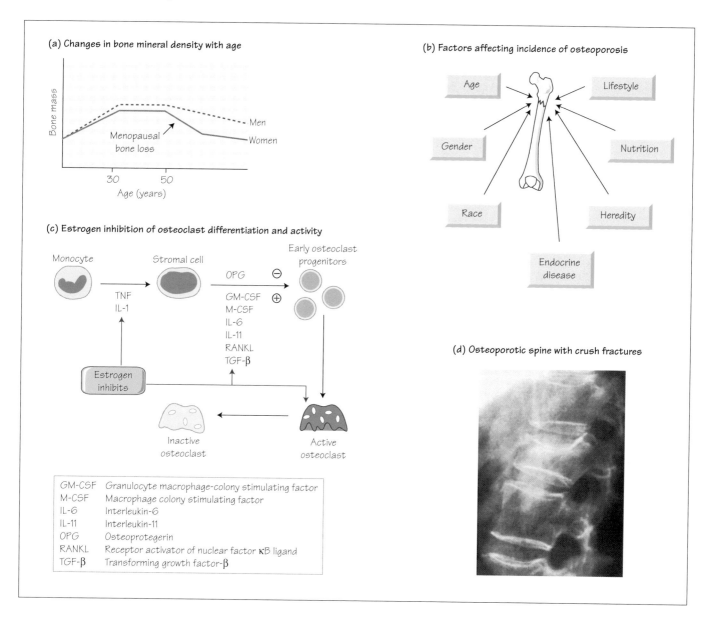

(a) Changes in bone mineral density with age

(b) Factors affecting incidence of osteoporosis

(c) Estrogen inhibition of osteoclast differentiation and activity

GM-CSF	Granulocyte macrophage-colony stimulating factor
M-CSF	Macrophage colony stimulating factor
IL-6	Interleukin-6
IL-11	Interleukin-11
OPG	Osteoprotegerin
RANKL	Receptor activator of nuclear factor κB ligand
TGF-β	Transforming growth factor-β

(d) Osteoporotic spine with crush fractures

Clinical background

Osteoporosis is a common disease of the elderly, affecting over 2 million women in the UK, and associated with significant morbidity and mortality. It is characterized by 'fragility fractures', defined as a fracture occurring after a fall from standing height or less and it is estimated that 33% of women and 20% of men over the age of 80 will sustain a hip fracture due to osteoporosis. Other common sites for osteoporotic fractures include the spine and distal radius (Colles' fracture) and it is estimated that the cost to the UK National Health Service and social services of treatment for osteoporotic fractures of the hip alone is in the order of £2.3 billion per annum. Primary

osteoporosis in women is due to a combination of age and estrogen deficiency; the cause in men is less clear but probably includes age-related falls in both estrogen and androgen concentrations.

Osteoporosis occurs in the context of lifetime changes in bone density. Peak bone density in both males and females is achieved in the late 20's and age-related bone loss begins at the start of the fifth decade. Peak bone mass is genetically determined and a major predictor of osteoporosis risk in later life. Other factors include sex hormone status, nutrition, calcium and vitamin D status and levels of physical activity. Both men and women exhibit age-related bone loss from the fifth decade, but the process in women is accelerated during the menopause, reflecting the role of estrogen as a major factor in the maintenance of bone mineral density. Osteoporosis is diagnosed by assessing bone mineral density by means of dual-energy X-ray absorptiometry (DEXA) scanning. The patient's score is measured according to standard deviation scores below normal peak bone mass.

A number of risk factors for osteoporosis have been identified and include age, sex, family history, Caucasian or Asian ethnicity, history of thyroid disease, cigarette smoking and excessive alcohol intake. The major risk factor for fractures in the elderly with osteoporosis is falling. Assessment of the patient should always include risk factors for falling such as visual impairment, cardiovascular disease with syncope, neuromuscular weakness and environmental hazards such as steps or poorly fitting carpets.

Therapeutic intervention may be offered as primary prevention to postmenopausal women, with significant risk factors depending upon their bone density and as secondary prevention following a fracture (see Chapter 55).

Aetiology

Osteoporosis is loss of bone mass and is the most common metabolic bone disease. Gender, race, heredity, lifestyle and nutrition, particularly the degree of calcium intake during the period of peak bone growth, determine the incidence of osteoporosis (Fig. 54b). The main phases of bone mass change are: (i) attainment of peak bone mass during postpubertal life and completion of bone mass consolidation between the ages of 20 and 30; (ii) commencement of bone loss between the ages of 30 and 40, which occurs equally in trabecular and cortical bone – approximately 25% of bone is lost; and (iii) postmenopausal loss of bone, mainly trabecular (e.g. vertebral), secondary to estrogen loss (Fig. 54a).

People of African Caribbean origin have, on average, a higher peak bone mass than other ethnic groups. Mother–daughter and twin studies suggest that hip fracture is more likely when there is a maternal history of osteoporosis, which may be accounted for by inheritance of polymorphic alleles of the vitamin D receptor gene in some populations. Nutritionally, an adequate intake of calcium by growing children and young adults is critical in the attainment of genetically determined peak bone mass, and calcium supplements have been shown to slow the rate of bone loss in the elderly, although it is not certain whether calcium supplements reduce the risk of fractures.

Exercise is an important factor in determining the rate of loss of bone mass with ageing in both men and women, and in both pre- and postmenopausal women. The risk of hip fractures may be reduced through regular exercise, although it is not clear whether this is due to maintenance of adequate bone density or to maintenance of agility, balance and muscle strength. Smoking has been shown to increase the rate of metabolism of exogenous estrogens (for example in oral contraceptives), although it is not known if smoking has this metabolic effect on endogenously produced estrogens. A history of thyrotoxicosis is a risk factor for osteoporosis.

Recent studies have found evidence that 5-HT in the gut slows or may even stop phosphate uptake in the gut. This is being actively studied and could conceivably generate novel treatments to supplement mainstream treatments of osteoporosis.

Estrogen and osteoporosis

Osteoporosis through estrogen deficiency is not age-dependent; accelerated bone loss may occur in hypogonadal women of whatever cause. After menopause, there is an acceleration of bone resorption due to estrogen deficiency, detected at biopsy as increased activation frequency of basic multicellular units on bone and increased resorption surfaces. There is increased excretion of metabolites of collagen and bone and a moderate depression of PTH secretion. The coupling mechanism of remodelling is maintained, with significant increases in levels of serum alkaline phosphatase, osteocalcin and bone-specific alkaline phosphatase. All these are indices of high bone turnover rates. Estrogen dampens osteoclast function partly through inhibition of monocyte activation and of osteoblast activity through suppression of genes that express IL-1, IL-6 and TNF (Fig. 54c).

The onset of osteoporosis is often painless and insidious and, unless routine bone scans are done, the first symptoms are due to the fracture. **Spinal fractures** in particular may be painless, or present as persistent back pain that is relieved by bed rest and exacerbated by any weight-bearing action (Fig. 54d). Fracture healing brings remission from pain. With multiple compression fractures of the spine a sharply localized forward angulation, called kyphosis, may result. The deformity is caused by collapse of the anterior section of the vertebra. Appendicular osteoporotic fractures (fractures of the limb bones) are often characterized by fractures of the distal radius and the femoral neck.

Imaging studies and laboratory findings

Bone densitometry is a reliable diagnostic tool. It measures the total bone density or calcium content at the wrist, spine and hip. The margin of error is small (1–2%) and the radiation dose administered is a fraction of that given by X-ray. Other methods include quantitative computed topography, which is more precise for cancellous than for compact bone. X-rays are used but are less sensitive and can give false positives since overpenetrated films may misrepresent a normal spine as osteopenic. Osteoporosis will not be detected by X-ray until approximately 35–55% of bone mass is lost.

Laboratory parameters

Osteocalcin and bone-specific alkaline phosphatase, markers of bone formation, may be raised. Hormonal indices in blood more often reflect age-related changes than any that might be associated with osteoporosis. Serum levels of $1,2,5(OH)_2D$ may be lower in patients with osteoporosis but this is more likely to be due to the reduction observed with ageing, and explained by reduced renal mass. Overall, serum chemistry values are normal in patients with osteoporosis. Alkaline phosphatase levels are raised when there is bone healing after osteoporotic fractures.

55 Metabolic bone disease: III Secondary osteoporosis

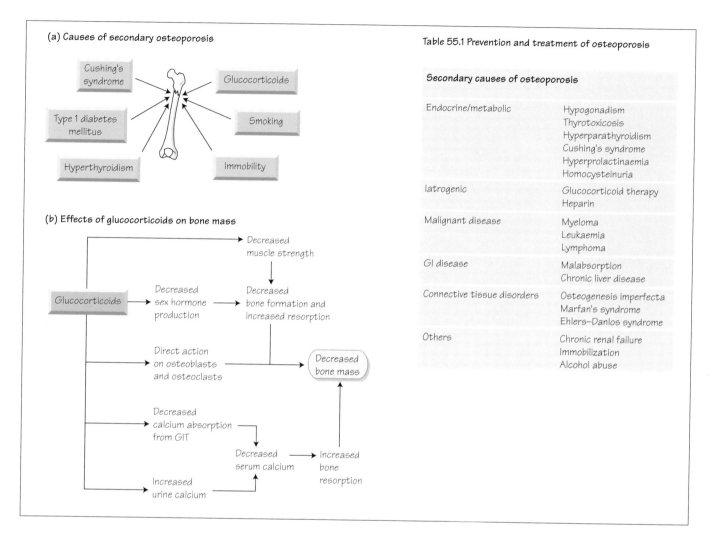

(a) Causes of secondary osteoporosis

Cushing's syndrome

Glucocorticoids

Type 1 diabetes mellitus

Smoking

Hyperthyroidism

Immobility

(b) Effects of glucocorticoids on bone mass

Glucocorticoids

Decreased muscle strength

Decreased sex hormone production → Decreased bone formation and increased resorption

Direct action on osteoblasts and osteoclasts

Decreased bone mass

Decreased calcium absorption from GIT

Increased urine calcium

Decreased serum calcium → Increased bone resorption

Table 55.1 Prevention and treatment of osteoporosis

Secondary causes of osteoporosis

Endocrine/metabolic	Hypogonadism
	Thyrotoxicosis
	Hyperparathyroidism
	Cushing's syndrome
	Hyperprolactinaemia
	Homocysteinuria
Iatrogenic	Glucocorticoid therapy
	Heparin
Malignant disease	Myeloma
	Leukaemia
	Lymphoma
GI disease	Malabsorption
	Chronic liver disease
Connective tissue disorders	Osteogenesis imperfecta
	Marfan's syndrome
	Ehlers–Danlos syndrome
Others	Chronic renal failure
	Immobilization
	Alcohol abuse

Introduction

Osteoporosis may occur as a secondary problem in patients with a range of endocrine and other disorders (Fig. 55a; Table 55.1). A high proportion of patients treated chronically with glucocorticoids develop osteoporosis. It may develop in patients immobilized for long periods, when bone resorption develops with consequent hypercalciuria and hypercalcaemia, especially in younger patients in whom bone turnover is normally rapid. Osteoporosis has been observed in astronauts, presumably due to the loss of gravitational effects, although the aetiology of this phenomenon is unknown. Hereditary disorders of collagen expression and metabolism may result in osteoporosis. These include Ehlers–Danlos syndrome, homocysteinuria and osteogenesis imperfecta.

The vast majority of patients with osteoporosis have the primary condition but causes of secondary osteoporosis should always be sought when undertaking clinical assessment.

Glucocorticoids and osteoporosis

Glucocorticoids, used to treat inflammatory disorders, cause osteoporosis, affecting predominantly the trabecular bone of the axial skeleton such that vertebral fractures are more common than those of the hip. Glucocorticoids cause osteoporosis through a wide variety of actions (Fig. 55b).

Direct actions. Glucocorticoids directly inhibit the replication of osteoblast lineages and the biosynthesis of new osteoblast cells and they induce apoptosis of osteoblasts, partially through their interactions with growth factors such as the insulin-like growth factors. In addition, glucocorticoids may directly decrease synthesis of osteocalcin, a component of bone matrix, and stimulate the synthesis of collagenase-3, which breaks down collagen types I and II, essential building blocks of bone. Furthermore, glucocorticoids stimulate osteoclast activity directly, and possibly indirectly, via secondary hyperparathyroidism.

Indirect actions. Glucocorticoids inhibit calcium absorption from the GIT and increase renal excretion, which may contribute to the development of secondary hyperparathyroidism. Glucocorticoids are associated with decreased plasma levels of estrogens and testosterone by suppressing adrenocorticotrophic hormone (ACTH) secretion from the anterior pituitary gland, thus resulting in suppression of adrenal androgen production. Luteinizing hormone production is decreased with consequent lowering of both estradiol and testosterone production in women and men respectively. Glucocorticoids also inhibit growth hormone production. Patients with Cushing's syndrome, which is associated with excessive adrenal activity, may also be at risk of osteoporosis and fractures.

Glucocorticoid therapy is a major cause of rapid bone loss and primary preventive therapy with bisphosphonates should be prescribed for every patient about to start a course of steroid therapy for more than 3 months.

Other endocrine disorders

Hyperthyroidism can cause osteoporosis by the direct action of thyroid hormone on bone resorption, since thyroid hormone is normally associated with high bone turnover. Fractures are uncommon in hyperthyroidism due to prompt diagnosis and treatment. Postmenopausal women with osteoporosis and a history of hyperthyroidism are, however, at increased risk of hip fractures. Type 1 diabetes mellitus is associated with mild osteopenia of cortical bone, although there does not seem to be a high incidence of fractures in these patients. Patients with Type 2 diabetes mellitus, on the other hand, usually have normal bone mass.

Heritable disorders

Several hundreds of mutations of the collagen Type 1 gene have been reported, some of which may result in defective osteoblast activity and result in brittle and fragile bones. Osteogenesis imperfecta, for example, is caused by a mutation of the gene which codes for Type 1 collagen, the main structural protein in bone matrix. Different phenotypes may produce anything from a relatively mild condition to one that is lethal to the embryo.

Immobilization and osteoporosis

Patients who are immobilized for prolonged periods, for example with neuromuscular disease or after spinal injuries, are risk of developing osteoporosis. Prolonged immobility in bed may reduce bone density by about 0.5% each month. Lumbar spine density may decrease at a rate of about 1% each week, resulting in anything up to a 50% loss of bone mass after a year. This is reversible, and mineralization of bone is initiated when the patient becomes ambulatory again.

Prevention and treatment of osteoporosis

Patients at risk from osteoporosis should be given suitable lifestyle advice to maintain adequate nutrition and normal body weight, to stop smoking and moderate excess alcohol intake and to take as much weight-bearing exercise as possible. Patients with established disease may benefit from hip-protectors if they are at risk of falling, plus suitable occupational therapy assessment and walking aids.

Estrogen replacement therapy at the menopause, with or without progestagens, has formed the mainstay of treatment in women to prevent postmenopausal bone loss. However, recent data from large observational studies have raised questions about the safety of HRT in women over 50 years in terms of the increased risk of breast cancer. Estrogen replacement should be offered to immediate women around the time of the menopause for symptomatic relief but it is no longer recommended as first-line therapy for the prevention of osteoporosis in women over 50 years. Younger women with premature ovarian failure continue to receive estrogen up to 50 years of age.

Therapeutic intervention as primary prevention may be offered to postmenopausal women with significant risk factors depending upon their bone density. The bisphosphonates etidronate, alendronate and risendronate have all been shown to prevent bone loss in the spine and hip, both in healthy women at the menopause and in older patients with established osteoporosis. Alendronate and risendronate have also both been shown to reduce the fracture rate in women with osteoporosis. Strontium ranelate may be offered to women intolerant of bisphosphonates. Following a fracture, the same drugs may be offered or alternatives such as raloxifene considered. Teriperatide, a PTH analogue, may be used where no other drug is tolerated or effective.

Glucocorticoid-induced osteoporosis should be prevented by primary prevention in patients starting treatment by the coprescription of a bisphosphonate. In patients who have been on prednisolone 7.5 mg daily or equivalent for 6 months or more, a dual emission X-ray absorptiometry (DEXA) scan will establish the bone mineral density and treatment can be given accordingly.

MCQs

There may be more than one correct answer for each question.

Chapter 1: Introduction

1 The principal endocrine glands include:
   (a) The salivary glands
   (b) Pituitary
   (c) The bile duct
   (d) The heart
   (e) The gut
2 Androgens:
   (a) Have mainly catabolic actions
   (b) Include dihydrotestosterone
   (c) Control tertiary sexual characteristics
   (d) Are secreted mainly from the testis and adrenal gland
   (e) Include DHEAS
3 The hypothalamo-pituitary portal blood system:
   (a) Carries neurohormones from the anterior and posterior pituitary to specific hypothalamic nuclei
   (b) Originates in the basal hypothalamic area
   (c) Is a major target for negative feedback control systems
   (d) Can be obstructed by tumour growth
   (e) Receives neurohormones from the brain for transport to the pituitary gland
4 The endocrine pancreas secretes:
   (a) Somatostatin
   (b) Inhibin
   (c) Insulin
   (d) Glucagon
   (e) Gastrin
5 Hormones secreted by the kidney include:
   (a) Renin
   (b) Vitamin D
   (c) Erythropoietin
   (d) Melatonin
   (e) Cholecystokinin

Chapter 2: Chemical transmission

1 In the classification of endocrine hormones:
   (a) Autocrine hormones act at cellular locations sites distal from their site of release
   (b) Autocrine hormones act on the cell which produces them
   (c) Paracrine hormones act on neighbouring cells
   (d) Endocrine hormones act on cells to which they are carried in one of the body's ductal systems
   (e) Neuroendocrine hormones are those that act only on neurones
2 Diffusion is:
   (a) The facilitated transport of molecules and ions through cell membranes
   (b) The movement of solutes in a fluid solvent
   (c) The active transport of solutes in a liquid phase
   (d) The decompression of a gas or liquid
   (e) The filtering of solutes
3 Facilitated transport:
   (a) Is the transport of chemicals across membranes by carrier proteins
   (b) Utilizes energy in the form of ATP
   (c) Albumin binds oestrogens specifically in blood
   (d) Utilizes carrier proteins
   (e) Osmosis is the movement of solutes across a semipermeable membrane from a region of low osmolarity to a higher one

Chapter 3: Mechanisms of hormone action: I Membrane receptors

1 Which of the following are true?
   (a) Charged ions diffuse freely through biological membranes
   (b) Hormones bind to receptors that recognize them selectively
   (c) When hormones bind to receptors it induces a conformational change in the hormone
   (d) Membrane receptors bind selectively to the nuclear membrane
   (e) Beta-blockers such as propranolol should not be used in asthma if possible

Chapter 4: Mechanisms of hormone action: II Intracellular receptors

1 Estrogen receptors:
   (a) Act principally on cell membrane-bound receptors to stimulate cyclic AMP activity
   (b) Are important targets for treatment of pancreatic cancer
   (c) Are members of the DNA-binding receptor super-family
   (d) Comprise two forms, viz. ER-α and er-β
   (e) In ovarian cancer, the β-form predominates
2 The thyroid:
   (a) The thyroid receptors are mainly cell membrane-bound
   (b) Thyroid receptors can bind DNA in the absence of the hormone leading, usually, to transcriptional repression
   (c) In the presence of the hormone, the receptors become transcriptional activators
   (d) To date, no isoforms of the thyroid receptor have been identified
   (e) The thyroid gland is situated just above the heart
3 Estrogen receptors are useful in that:
   (a) They are predictive for treatment choices in breast cancer
   (b) They are used to predict female fertility status
   (c) Their identification has yielded clinical treatments, for example, tamoxifen
   (d) They are targets for treatment of postpartum depression
   (e) Their distribution increases knowledge of sites of estrogen action

Chapter 5: The hypothalamus and pituitary gland

1 A pituitary tumour could cause:
  (a) Bilateral blindness
  (b) Hyperprolactinaemia
  (c) Unusual fatigue
  (d) Syncope
  (e) Exuberant hair growth
2 The hypothalamus:
  (a) Lies at the base of the brain below the pituitary gland
  (b) Contains the supraoptic nuclei which send axons to the anterior pituitary
  (c) Has a medial nucleus that communicates with other brain areas mainly via the medial forebrain bundle
  (d) Is essential for maintenance of sexual function through GnRH
  (e) Medial eminence is where neurohormones join the vascular link with the anterior pituitary gland
3 Hypothalamic neurohormones include:
  (a) Thyroid-stimulating hormone
  (b) Gonadotrophin-releasing hormone
  (c) Prolactin
  (d) Thyrotrophin-releasing hormone
  (e) GHRH
4 The pituitary gland:
  (a) Is also termed the hypophysis
  (b) Consists, mainly, of two subglands
  (c) The anterior lobe is called the neuohypophysis
  (d) Communicates with the brain by means of both portal blood and neural links

Chapter 6: Gonadotrophin-releasing hormone: a peptide hormone

1 Gonadotrophin-releasing hormone (GnRH):
  (a) Is released in a pulsatile fashion
  (b) Is released into the general circulation
  (c) Causes release of the pituitary gonadotrophins LH and FSH
  (d) Binds to intracellular pituitary receptors for GnRH
  (e) Deficiency causes infertility
2 Synthesis and release of GnRH:
  (a) Initially involves the translation of the gene that codes for GnRH
  (b) Requires activation by an initiation site upstream from the coding region
  (c) Is triggered by the neurotransmitter norepinephrine
  (d) May be physiologically inhibited by opioids
  (e) Is a target for treatment of infertility
3 Exocytosis:
  (a) Is a cellular mechanism for hormone release
  (b) Initially involves a fall in intracellular levels of cyclic AMP
  (c) Requires a rise in intracellular free Ca^{2+}
  (d) Is facilitated by relaxation of cellular microfilaments
  (e) Achieves transfer of GnRH into the portal blood system

Chapter 7: Principles of feedback control

1 Homeostasis:
  (a) Involves the maintenance of fluid, salt and hormone balance
  (b) Does not require the integration of neural, biochemical and physical systems
  (c) Requires signals, transducers, sensors and responders
  (d) Involves the coordinated actions of enzymes and receptors
  (e) Within hormonal systems is independent of hormone levels
2 A positive feedback system:
  (a) Amplifies the subsequent response of a hormonal or neural output system
  (b) Is an integral mechanism in the successful inhibition of ovulation
  (c) Results in the LH surge and ovulation
  (d) Inhibits or reduces further release of the hormone
  (e) Is the mechanism of action of oral contraceptives

Chapter 8: Endocrine function tests

1 Which of the following may affect the interpretation of single hormone measurements?
  (a) High carbohydrate diet
  (b) Pulsatile secretion
  (c) Stress
  (d) Temperature of the sample
  (e) Time of measurement
2 The insulin tolerance test:
  (a) Includes serial measurements of ACTH
  (b) Is required to demonstrate GH deficiency
  (c) May be replaced by the short synacthen test in patients with ischaemic heart disease
  (d) Should not be performed if the patient has epilepsy
  (e) Tests the response to a hyperglycaemic stimulus

Chapter 9: Growth: I Cellular growth factors

1 The cell cycle:
  (a) Involves an initial synthetic phase (S), which prepares the cell for the growth phase G_1
  (b) The M phase is the splitting of the parent cell into two daughter cells
  (c) New cells may remain in the G_o phase, e.g. neurones or muscle cells
  (d) G_1-phase cells never enter the synthetic stage
  (e) Tumour cells may remain in GO before re-entering G_1
2 Growth factors, including some hormones:
  (a) Insulin-like growth factors do not mediate the action of growth hormone
  (b) Growth hormone (GH) mediates the release of IGF-1 and IGF-2 from the liver
  (c) Insulin is a catabolic hormone
  (d) Without insulin, amino acid uptake into tissues is inhibited
  (e) Without insulin, protein catabolism is enhanced
3 Nerve growth factor (NGF):
  (a) Is similar in structure to glucagon
  (b) Is secreted in large amounts by the submandibular gland
  (c) Thyroxine, testosterone and tri-iodothyronine are involved in control of NGF release
  (d) Binds to intracellular receptors to trigger de novo protein synthesis
  (e) Is critically involved in normal development of the nervous system

4 Epidermal growth factor (EGF):
(a) Was originally isolated from the mouse salivary gland
(b) Normally is associated with an IGF-binding protein
(c) Is released by α–adrenergic antagonists
(d) Promotes proliferation of epidermal cells
(e) Is present in breast milk as a mitogenic factor

5 Transforming growth factors:
(a) Include TGF-α and TGF-β
(b) Both inhibit fibroblast growth
(c) TGF-β may stimulate or inhibit cell growth
(d) TGF-β is pleiomorphic – at least five forms exist
(e) TGF-β has structural homology with inhibin

6 Platelet-derived growth factor (PDGF):
(a) Is synthesized and stored in blood platelets
(b) Is released when platelets are activated during cellular injury
(c) Has only one receptor
(d) Consists of a single, circularized peptide chain
(e) Is synthesized only by platelets

Chapter 10: Growth: II Normal growth

1 Causes of growth hormone deficiency (GHD) include:
(a) Cranial irradiation
(b) Perinatal trauma
(c) Dietary deficiency
(d) Anaemia
(e) Congenital midline structural defects of the hypothalamus

2 Features of GHD include:
(a) Growth failure
(b) Premature ageing of facial features
(c) Reduced muscle bulk
(d) Increased central fat deposition
(e) Reduced final height if untreated

3 Normal growth:
(a) Prenatally is independent of maternal diet
(b) Postnatally, is independent of social status
(c) Postnatally, is influenced by chronic disease
(d) Postanatally, there is good sex-specific correlation between child and parent height
(e) Is dependent on growth hormone/insulin-like growth factors

Chapter 11: Growth: III Growth hormone

1 Patients with GH deficiency (GHD):
(a) Have, as adults, marked physiological but not psychological problems
(b) Have decreased risk of heart disease
(c) Have increased atheroma risk
(d) Have decreased bone mineral density
(e) Are treated with daily SC injections of recombinant human GH

2 Which of the following are true?
(a) GH is synthesized in the somatotroph cells of the posterior pituitary gland
(b) GH has high structural homology with prolactin
(c) GH and prolactin share a single ancestral gene
(d) GH exists in the circulation in only one form
(e) GH consists of 91 amino acids

3 *Direct* actions of GH include:
(a) Lipolysis of adipocytes
(b) Bone growth
(c) Increased glucose production by liver and muscle
(d) A diabetogenic action
(e) Stimulation of IGF-1 production

4 Indirect actions of GH include:
(a) Stimulation of IGF-1 production
(b) Stimulation of lipolysis
(c) Inhibition of protein synthesis
(d) An anti-diabetic action
(e) Stimulation of cyclic AMP production

5 The growth hormone receptor:
(a) Consists of two domains, intracellular and extracellular
(b) Is member of a haematopoietic Type I cytokine receptor family
(c) Consists of two homologous domains
(d) Triggers intracellular cyclic AMP synthesis
(e) Mediates intracellular JAK2 recruitment

Chapter 12: Growth: IV Pathophysiology

1 Excess GH secretion is due primarily to:
(a) A pituitary adenoma
(b) Peripheral GHRH-secreting adenomas
(c) The MEN syndrome
(d) Drug abuse
(e) The contraceptive pill.

2 Clinical features of acromegaly include:
(a) Carpal tunnel syndrome
(b) Hypotension
(c) Prognathism
(d) Sweating
(e) Paraesthesiae

Chapter 13: Thyroid: I Thyroid gland and thyroid hormones

1 The thyroid gland:
(a) Is situated posteriorly in the neck
(b) Function is production and release of the one hormone thyroxin (T_4)
(c) Produces thyroid hormones essential for normal development
(d) Has the parathyroid glands embedded within it
(e) Begins to develop within two weeks after conception

2 During thyroid hormone biosynthesis:
(a) The thyroid-trapping mechanism pumps organic iodine into the cell
(b) Thyroglobulin is synthesized in the colloid
(c) Thyroglobulin binds iodine in the colloid
(d) One thyroglobulin molecule can bind up to four iodine residues
(e) Iodide uptake inhibitors include iodide ions

3 Thyroid stimulating hormone (TSH):
(a) Stimulates uptake of inorganic iodide
(b) Stimulates thyroglobulin synthesis
(c) Stimulates thyroglobulin-iodide complex reuptake from colloid
(d) Stimulates release of T_3 and T_4 from thyroglobulin
(e) Stimulates release of T_3 and T_4 into the circulation

4 During release and metabolism of T_3 and T_4:
   (a) The ratio of T_3/T_4 release is about 20 : 1
   (b) Most bioactive T_3 is derived through metabolism of T_4
   (c) Iodide released after metabolism of thyroid hormones excreted in faeces
   (d) The half-life of T3 in the circulation is shorter than that of T_4
   (e) T_3 is more potent than is T_4

Chapter 14: Thyroid: II Thyroid hormone secretion and action

1 In the developed world:
   (a) Most cases of hypothyroidism are due to insufficient dietary iodine
   (b) Hypothyroidism may be associated with destructive antithyroid antibodies
   (c) TSH receptor antibodies can cause hyperthyroid goitre
   (d) Hypothyroidism can be drug-induced, e.g. by lithium
   (e) Secondary hypothyroidism is relatively rare in general medical practice
2 TRH:
   (a) Is a tripeptide synthesized in the anterior pituitary gland
   (b) Is transported in the hypothalamus-anterior pituitary portal system
   (c) Stimulates de novo TSH synthesis in the anterior pituitary gland
   (d) Hypothalamic lesions may impair synthesis and release
   (e) Is stored in the median eminence
3 TSH:
   (a) Is the acronym for thyroid-stimulating hormone
   (b) Shares some structural homology with placental hCG
   (c) Is used clinically for thyroid function tests
   (d) The TSH gene is directly inhibited by T_3
   (e) TSH receptor antibodies do not affect thyroid function
4 Thyroid hormone:
   (a) Generates calorigenesis through stimulation of mitochondrial oxygen consumption
   (b) Inhibits intestinal absorption of glucose
   (c) Stimulates hepatic glycogenolysis
   (d) Inhibits insulin breakdown
   (e) Potentiates the glycogenolytic actions of epinephrine
5 During growth and development:
   (a) Fetal thyroid hormone is of maternal origin
   (b) The fetal thyroid is differentiated at about the 10th–11th week of gestation
   (c) Thyroid hormone is essential for normal fetal growth
   (d) Fetal hypothyroidism retards normal brain and skeletal development
   (e) Thyroid hormone is essential for normal growth hormone production

Chapter 15: Thyroid: III Thyroid pathophysiology

1 In hyperthyroidism:
   (a) Most cases are due to autoimmune thyrotoxicosis
   (b) Amiodarone may be a cause
   (c) There is marked weight gain
   (d) There is, frequently, noticeable bradycardia
   (e) Oedema

2 Thyrotoxicosis:
   (a) May be treated with antithyroid drugs
   (b) May be a symptom of autoimmune disease
   (c) May cause pre-tibial myxoedema
   (d) Rarely causes fatigue
   (e) Is associated with elevated serum TSH
3 Features of Graves' disease include:
   (a) Dry eyes
   (b) Exophthalmos
   (c) Chemosis (oedema of the conjunctiva)
   (d) Thyroid acropathy (digit clubbing)
   (e) Enhanced visual acuity

Chapter 16: Adrenal gland: I Adrenal medulla

1 Phaeochromocytomas:
   (a) Are tumours of the adrenal cortex
   (b) Secrete catecholamines
   (c) Are mainly malignant
   (d) Occur mainly in the adrenal medulla
   (e) Occur mainly in extramedullary locations
2 Catecholamines:
   (a) Are stored in granules in the adrenal cortex
   (b) Are metabolized intracellularly by monoamine oxidase
   (c) Actions are terminated by monoamine oxidase
   (d) Are taken up presynaptically by cells that release them
   (e) Are excreted in urine
3 Norepinephrine:
   (a) Is commonly known as the hormone of flight or fight
   (b) Is the immediate precursor of epinephrine
   (c) Is secreted by the adrenal medulla
   (d) Feeds back on α-2 receptors to limit its release
   (e) Is formed from dopamine
4 Actions of epinephrine include:
   (a) Increased heart rate and force through activation of β-1 receptors
   (b) Dilation of the pupil
   (c) Decreasing coagulation time
   (d) Bronchodilation
   (e) Constriction of cutaneous blood vessels

Chapter 17: Adrenal gland: II Adrenocortical hormones

1 Clinical features of Cushing's Syndrome include:
   (a) Hirsutism
   (b) Osteoporosis
   (c) Hypotension
   (d) Mania
   (e) Poor wound healing
2 The principal adrenocortical hormones in humans are:
   (a) Corticosterone
   (b) Aldosterone
   (c) Dehydroepiandrosterone sulphate
   (d) 27-hydroxyprogesterone
   (e) Epinephrine
3 Low density lipoprotein:
   (a) Protects against atherosclerotic disease
   (b) Transports cholesterol in the circulation
   (c) Has an inner core of cholesterol esters

(d) Is associated with Type III lipoproteinaemia

(e) Is also known as HDL

4 During biosynthesis of adrenocortical steroids:

(a) Adrenal androgens are synthesized from androstenedione

(b) Which is formed from 17-hydroxyprogrsterone

(c) Estrogens are formed through aromatization of the A ring

(d) Aromatization including the creation of alternating double bonds in the A ring of the steroid nucleus and:

(e) The removal of the methyl group at C19

Chapter 18: Adrenal gland: III Adrenocorticotrophic hormone (ACTH)

1 Symptoms of Cushing's Syndrome may include:

(a) Dry facial skin

(b) Acne

(c) Depression

(d) Facial hirsutism

(e) Elevated free urinary cortisol levels

2 ACTH:

(a) Is synthesized in the intermediate lobe of the pituitary gland

(b) Release is promoted by hypothalamic corticotrophin-releasing hormone (CRH)

(c) Activates target cells by activating the adenylate cyclase second messenger system

(d) Causes release of adrenocortical steroids

(e) Is released from the anterior pituitary gland

3 CRH:

(a) Is the acronym for cortisol-releasing hormone

(b) Release is stimulated by acetylcholine and 5-HT

(c) Contains 41 amino acids

(d) Stimulates IL-1 production

(e) Closes voltage-gated Ca^{2+} channels

Chapter 19: Adrenal gland: IV Cortisol and androgens

1 In congenital adrenal hyperplasia:

(a) Most cases are due to deficiencies in the 17-hydroxylase enzyme

(b) Androgen production may be significantly increased

(c) There may be ambiguous genitalia at birth

(d) In male babies there may be failure to thrive

(e) Treatment is usually with anti-androgens

2 Physiological actions of cortisol include:

(a) Inhibition of glucose uptake in muscle

(b) Initiation of parturition in humans

(c) Stimulation biosynthesis of enzymes that catalyse gluconeogenesis

(d) Breakdown of muscle to mobilize energy

(e) Feedback inhibition of ACTH release

3 Permissive actions of cortisol include:

(a) Facilitation of catecholamine synthesis and tissue uptake

(b) Inhibition of catecholamine-stimulated fat mobilization

(c) Body temperature maintenance

(d) Body's response to stress

(e) Memory recall

4 The general adaptation syndrome:

(a) Is generally abbreviated to GAS

(b) Is initiated by an alarm reaction, followed by:

(c) Resistance and then by:

(d) Renewal

Chapter 20: Adrenal gland: V Aldosterone

1 Aldosterone:

(a) Is synthesized in the zona reticularis of the adrenal cortex

(b) Synthesis includes the hydroxylation of corticosterone

(c) Secretion is controlled by the renin-angiotensin system

(d) Stimulates the active transport of K^+ through the epithelial cell wall

(e) Enhances Na+ transport through the epithelial cell wall of the kidney distal tubule

2 Aldosterone action may be through:

(a) Increasing Na^+ channels in apical membranes

(b) Increasing Na^+/K^{+-}ATPase molecules

(c) Inhibition of fatty acid biosynthesis

(d) Potentiation of acetylcholine action

(e) Alteration of membrane phospholipid composition

3 A patient with an adrenal adenoma may present with the following symptoms:

(a) Hypotension

(b) Left ventricular hypertrophy

(c) Hypokalaemia

(d) Elevated serum aldosterone levels

(e) Suppressed rennin activity

Chapter 21: Adrenal gland: VI Pathophysiology

1 Adrenocortical insufficiency:

(a) Presents as primary renal failure when the pathology originates in the adrenal gland

(b) Symptoms may include hypotension and

(c) reduced pigmentation of skin

(d) Hypertensive crisis

(e) Presence of adrenal autoantibodies

2 Causes of adrenal failure include:

(a) Autoimmune reactions

(b) Mutations of CRH receptors

(c) HIV/AIDS

(d) Metastatic tumours

(e) Adrenal hyperplasia

3 Hypoaldosteronism:

(a) Is an excess of aldosterone secretion

(b) Results in Na^+ loss

(c) Occurs in diabetes

(d) May be secondary to deficient rennin release

(e) Occurs occasionally because of aldosterone receptor defects in target cells

Chapter 22: Endocrine autoimmunity

1 Autoimmunity:

(a) May be defined as an attack on the host tissues by a foreign protein

(b) May occur as a temporary immune reaction or develop to become a chronic disease

(c) May be organ-specific or systemic

(d) Occurs seldom in women

(e) Attacks only anatomically close tissues

2 Hashimoto's thyroiditis:

(a) Does not damage the thyroid gland

(b) Occurs through development of autoantibodies to thyroid tissues

(c) Is more prevalent in women

(d) Is a direct antibody-mediated autoimmune disease

(e) Is a T-cell-mediated autoimmune disease

3 Graves' disease:

(a) Attacks several different endocrine organs

(b) Affects the adrenal gland

(c) Results in protruding eyeballs

(d) Is caused by excess thyroid hormone secretion

(e) Is not an example of an autoimmune disease

4 In immune-complex-mediated diseases:

(a) Diseases such as SLE are most probably caused by immune complex-mediated reactions

(b) There is probably no genetic input to the aetiology

(c) There are often circulating antibodies to cytoplasmic and nuclear factors

(d) The cytoplasmic and nuclear antigens themselves are always pathogenic

(e) Deposition of immune complexes in kidneys is a serious consequence of autoimmune disease

5 Regarding the role of sex hormones:

(a) There appears to be no sexual dimorphism in the occurrence of autoimmune endocrinopathies

(b) Remission of rheumatoid arthritis during pregnancy supports a sexual dimorphism in the occurrence of certain autoimmune diseases

(c) Systemic lupus erythematosus is equally distributed between the sexes

(d) Rheumatoid arthritis is more prevalent in women

(e) Rheumatoid arthritis and SLE are known to flare at puberty or after parturition

Chapter 23: Sexual differentiation and development: I Introduction

1 Sexually, every normally developed human has:

(a) 23 pairs of chromosomes in each cell

(b) If female, the normal karyotype is XX

(c) If male, the normal karyotype is XY

(d) Functionally normal testes producing spermatozoa

(e) If female, the XXY karyotope

2 During normal development of the male:

(a) The Sry antigen directs migration of primordial germ cells away from the medullary region of the primitive gonad

(b) Under Sry influence, the indifferent gonad begins to develop into a testis

(c) Primitive sex cords give rise to the seminiferous tubules

(d) The epithelial cells of the seminiferous tubules give rise to the germinal epithelium

(e) The epithelial cells also give rise to the Leydig cells

3 During normal development of the female:

(a) In the absence of the Sry antigen, the female gonads will not develop

(b) The XX karyotype is essential for normal sexual development

(c) The Müllerian ducts develop

(d) The external genitalia require maternal estrogen for development

(e) The genital tubercle will become the clitoris

4 Turner's Syndrome:

(a) Is a genetic mutation when there is usually only one X chromosome

(b) Produces a wide range of responses

(c) Does not occur in males

(d) In girls may be treated with low dose ethynylestradiol and growth hormone

(e) May stunt growth

5 In Kleinfelter's Syndrome:

(a) There are three sex chromosomes XXY

(b) May cause feminization in males

(c) Growth is always stunted

(d) There is no effect on hair growth and distribution

(e) May cause breast growth in males

Chapter 24: Sexual differentiation and development: II Puberty

1 The timing and onset of puberty:

(a) Is independent of genetic factors

(b) Is dependent on body weight and composition

(c) Is at an earlier age in Eastern civilizations

(d) Is marked by a rise in the secretion of LH

(e) And a rise in sex hormone secretion

2 Hormonal changes at or around the onset of puberty include:

(a) A fall in growth hormone secretion

(b) Pulsatile release of growth hormone

(c) Leptin signalling to the hypothalamus regarding body weight changes

(d) Establishment of 90-minute pulses of LH secretion

(e) Establishment of evening peaks of testosterone in boys

3 Delayed puberty:

(a) Is defined as absence of breast development in girls by 13:5 years, and

(b) In boys, failure of testicular growth to >4 ml by 14 years

(c) Is due to pulsatile release of GnRH

(d) Is a common referral to paediatricians

(e) In boys can be treated with low-dose testosterone

Chapter 25: Female reproduction: I Menstrual cycle

1 The female reproductive organs:

(a) Include the ovaries, fallopian tubes, uterus and vagina

(b) Principal roles include the activation of sperm

(c) Produce and prepare the ovum for fertilization

(d) Prepare the uterus for implantation

(e) Provide a benign host for the development of the fetus

2 During the menstrual cycle:

(a) As a safety precaution, several follicles develop fully

(b) FSH promotes follicle development

(c) LH stimulates estrogen production

(d) LH promotes LH receptor proliferation

(e) Inhibin suppresses FSH secretion

3 Estrogen actions during the menstrual cycle include:
  (a) Glandular proliferation in the uterine endothelium
  (b) Suppression of progesterone receptor biosynthesis
  (c) Proliferation of vaginal epithelium
  (d) Negative feedback on LH release
  (e) Inhibition of the pre-ovulatory LH surge

4 At maturation of the Graafian follicle:
  (a) Progesterone secretion increases
  (b) An LH surge into the bloodstream occurs
  (c) This surge inhibits ovum release
  (d) The corpus luteum is transferred into a Graafian follicle
  (e) If fertilization occurs, the corpus luteum atrophies and no further progesterone is released

5 Clinical monitoring of the menstrual cycle:
  (a) May be useful when assessing sub-fertility
  (b) Involves monitoring of cycle dates
  (c) And symptoms of mid-cycle lower abdominal pain and increased cervical secretion
  (d) May include ultrasound scanning for possible ovulatory disorders
  (e) As well as tracking progesterone release

Chapter 26: Female reproduction: II Ovarian steroids

1 Polycystic ovary syndrome:
  (a) Is the commonest cause of hirsutism and irregular cycles
  (b) Is associated with atrophied ovaries
  (c) Has symptoms suggesting raised circulating testosterone levels
  (d) Does not affect the menstrual cycle
  (e) Should be treated to lower circulating androgens

2 Physiological effects of estrogens in reproduction include:
  (a) Sexual differentiation of the female genitalia and accessory sex organs
  (b) Stimulation of breast and vaginal development during puberty
  (c) Closure of the epiphyses
  (d) Maintenance of the menstrual cycle
  (e) Prevention of fluid retention in pregnancy

3 Metabolic actions of estrogens include:
  (a) Inhibition of bone resorption
  (b) Increasing bowel motility
  (c) Stimulation of SHBG production by the liver
  (d) Increasing levels of high-density lipoproteins (HDL)
  (e) Increase platelet aggregation

4 Estrogen's main mechanism of action involves:
  (a) Initial binding to a cell surface receptor
  (b) Three isoforms of the receptor, viz. α, β and π
  (c) Initial binding to intracellular protein receptors
  (d) Transcriptional activation
  (e) *De novo* protein synthesis

5 Ovarian androgens:
  (a) Are important local regulators of ovarian function
  (b) Are aromatized in theca cells
  (c) In excess interfere with normal reproductive function
  (d) Include androstenedione and testosterone
  (e) Are produced in the granulosa cells of the ovary

Chapter 27: Female reproduction: III Pregnancy

1 Fertilization is:
  (a) The mitotic division of the zygote
  (b) The formation of the early blastocyst
  (c) The formation of the trophoblast
  (d) The fusion of ovum and sperm pronuclei
  (e) Acceptance of the blastocyst by the endometrial epithelium

2 If the ovum is fertilized and implanted:
  (a) The corpus luteum continues to secret estradiol
  (b) The syncytiotrophoblast continues to secrete hCG
  (c) The corpus luteum synthesizes relaxin, which:
  (d) Relaxes abdominal muscle
  (e) The placenta attains maturity by the end of the first trimester

3 Steroid actions during pregnancy include:
  (a) Enhancement of uterine motility by progesterone
  (b) Progesterone-induced decrease of uterine sensitivity to oxytocin
  (c) A soporific effect of estradiol
  (d) Rising blood levels of estriol as an index of normal fetal development
  (e) Estrogen-mediated rise in maternal plasma prolactin levels

Chapter 28: Female reproduction: IV Parturition and lactation

1 Factors possibly involved in the stimulation and initiation of parturition include:
  (a) Falling estrogen levels
  (b) An increase in uterine oxytocin receptors
  (c) Rapid fetal growth
  (d) Maturation of the hypothalamo-pituitary system
  (e) A rapid fall in fetal cortisol blood levels

2 Important chemical and mechanical mechanisms implicated in initiating parturition include:
  (a) The growing size of the fetus
  (b) Increased production of PG_{E2} and $PF\alpha$
  (c) Decreased intracellular Ca^{2+}
  (d) Fall in intracellular cAMP levels
  (e) Increased activity of inflammatory mediators

3 Important stimulants and mechanisms of lactation include:
  (a) A sustained fall in prolactin levels
  (b) Growth of the mammary lobular-alveolar system
  (c) A fall in estrogen and progesterone activity
  (d) Activation of the phospholipase A_2 second messenger system
  (e) Increased prostaglandin synthesis

4 In the mediation of the suckling reflex:
  (a) Suckling generates a reflex inhibition of oxytocin release from the posterior pituitary gland
  (b) Dopamine exerts an inhibitory effect on prolactin release
  (c) The neurotransmitter GABA increases prolactin activity
  (d) Angiotensin II stimulates the lactotrophs
  (e) Suckling promotes fertility in the mother

5 The role of the brain in controlling suckling may include:
  (a) The activity of a neural prolactin-releasing peptide
  (b) A stimulant activity of thyrotrophin-releasing hormone

(c) An inhibitory action of angiotensin

(d) Stress

(e) Lactation-produced infertility

Chapter 29: Female reproduction: V Pathophysiology

1 Primary amenorrhoea:
   (a) Is defined as the absence of menses by 16 years
   (b) Is the most common menstrual disorder
   (c) May be caused by disorders of genital differentiation
   (d) May be caused by irradiation
   (e) May be a result of delayed puberty

2 Hypothalamic-pituitary disease:
   (a) May result from radio/chemotherapy
   (b) Psychological disorders
   (c) May be the result of a tumour
   (d) May reflect combined pituitary hormone deficiencies
   (e) Often results from excess corticotrophin release

3 Hypothalamic amenorrhoea:
   (a) Treatment should include an intensive fitness-training regime
   (b) Is most frequently caused by anterior pituitary tumours
   (c) Is the commonest cause of secondary amenorrhoea seen in endocrine clinics
   (d) Treatment aims most importantly include weight gain and reduced exercise activity
   (e) If left untreated could result in osteoporosis

4 Polycystic ovary syndrome (PCOS):
   (a) May result from androgen- or estrogen-secreting tumours
   (b) Usually produces oligomenorrhoea and other signs of androgen excess
   (c) Patients may present with symptoms of hypoinsulinaemeia
   (d) Often produces weight loss
   (e) Treatment should include active exercise programmes and weight reduction

Chapter 30: Female reproduction: VI Contraception

1 Relatively reliable contraception choices include:
   (a) The rhythm method
   (b) Combined oral contraceptives (COC)
   (c) Hypnosis
   (d) Postcoital contraception
   (e) Progestogen-only contraceptives

2 The combined oral contraceptive:
   (a) Is presently the most reliable form of COC
   (b) Contains two doses of a potent progestogen
   (c) Is contraindicated in women with a history of cardiovascular disease
   (d) Prevents ovulation through positive feedback on gonadotrophin secretion
   (e) May also act directly on the uterus and cervix

3 Progestogen-only pills:
   (a) Were introduced to avoid the adverse effects of estrogen-containing OCs
   (b) Act mainly by thinning the vaginal mucus
   (c) Are more reliable than are OCs

(d) Increase low-density lipoproteins in plasma

(e) Cause abnormal responses to glucose tolerance tests

Chapter 31: Male reproduction: I The testis

1 The major mechanism of androgen action is:
   (a) Through cell membrane-bound androgen receptors
   (b) Inhibition of estrogen receptors
   (c) Initial binding to intracellular androgen receptor proteins
   (d) For androgenic actions, initial conversion to 5-α-dihydrotestosterone
   (e) Through activation of the inositol second messenger system

2 Normal fertility in the male is achieved through:
   (a) Adequate nutrition
   (b) The production of healthy and vigorously motile spermatozoa
   (c) Adequate testosterone production by the Leydig cells
   (d) Adequate FSH release for normal testicular development
   (e) Healthy exercise

3 Normal testicular function depends on:
   (a) Pulsatile release of GnRH to the anterior pituitary gland
   (b) Adequate release of LH and FSH from the anterior pituitary gland
   (c) Crucial stimulation of testicular FSH receptors by prolactin
   (d) Normal production of 17-ketosteroids
   (e) Stimulation of FSH release by inhibin

4 Biosynthesis of testosterone:
   (a) Takes place in the Sertoli cell
   (b) Is promoted by FSH
   (c) Involves the initial conversion of pregnenolone to cholesterol
   (d) Includes the 17-hydroxylation of pregnenolone
   (e) The conversion of 17-keosteroids to testosterone

5 Key reactions in the mechanism and action of testosterone include:
   (a) Initial high affinity binding reaction with a cell membrane-bound androgen receptor
   (b) Conversion to the active metabolite 5-α-dihydrotestosterone (DHT)
   (c) Translocation of the androgen-receptor complex to the nucleus
   (d) *De novo* protein synthesis
   (e) Excretion of testosterone in the urine

Chapter 32: Male reproduction: II Actions of androgens

1 Causes of hypogonadotropic hypogonadism in the male include:
   (a) GnRH receptor mutations
   (b) Weight gain
   (c) Anabolic steroids
   (d) Pituitary tumours
   (e) Head injuries

2 Actions of androgens include:
   (a) Sexual differentiation of the mammalian brain
   (b) Maintenance of spermatogenesis
   (c) Decreasing red blood cell production

(d) Inhibition of the actions of FSH

(e) Increases basal metabolic rate

3 Failure or absence of androgen action may result in:

(a) Hypogonadotropic hypogonadism

(b) Delayed or failed puberty in boys

(c) Failed libido

(d) Loss of appetite

(e) Sub-fertility

Chapter 33: Male reproduction: III Pathophysiology

1 Primary seminiferous tubule failure:

(a) May result from chemotherapy in childhood

(b) Always results in atrophied testes

(c) Reduces testosterone production

(d) Results in untreatable infertility

(e) Androgen replacement therapy may be considered

2 Male gynaecomastia:

(a) Is breast enlargement in males

(b) Is usually caused by excess weight-lifting exercises

(c) When accompanied by galactorrhoea, maybe indicative of excess prolactin secretion

(d) In ageing men may be indicative of an increased circulating androgen/estrogen ratio

(e) May occur with regular use of cannabis

3 Impotence:

(a) Is loss of libido

(b) Is mainly of endocrine origin

(c) May result from reduced blood supply to the penis, thus preventing erection

(d) Can be treated with sildenafil (Viagra)

(e) Viagra blocks phosphodiesterase-5

4 Benign prostatic hyperplasia (BPH):

(a) Is growth of the lateral lobes of the prostate gland in middle-aged men

(b) May result in occlusion of the urethra

(c) Is delayed by continued androgen production and release

(d) Should not be treated with surgery

(e) Can be treated with aromatase inhibitors

5 Prostatic cancer:

(a) Is almost always androgen-dependent

(b) Treatment aims at complete ablation of the tumour and removal of all sources of androgen production in the body

(c) Can be treated with stable analogues of GnRH

(d) And with androgen receptor antagonists

(e) NB: When starting GnRH treatment, an androgen receptor antagonist should be administered with the first doses to block the effects of an initial, transient surge of testosterone production

Chapter 34: Oxytocin

1 Oxytocin:

(a) Is a nonapeptide produced by and released from the anterior pituitary gland

(b) Induces contraction of the uterine smooth muscle 2–3 weeks before parturition

(c) Receptors activate the intracellular PLC/IP3 system in target cells

(d) Inhibits maternal behaviour

(e) Release is inhibited by stress

2 Oxytocin biosynthesis and secretion:

(a) Oxytocin biosynthesis occurs in the cell bodies of the magnocellular neurones of the paraventricular and supraoptic nuclei

(b) Reaches the posterior pituitary via the axons from the brain that terminate in close contact with capillaries in the posterior pituitary gland

(c) Oxytocin activates mainly the cAMP second messenger system

(d) Oxytocin elicits only male sexual behaviour

(e) Oxytocin inhibits milk ejection from the breast.

Chapter 35: Vasopressin

1 Vasopressin:

(a) Is an octapeptide synthesized only in the hypothalamus

(b) Has a powerful diuretic action

(c) Lack will cause diabetes insipidus

(d) Has no significant physiological action on blood pressure

(e) Is expressed in virtually all cell types in the body

2 Causes of diabetes insipidus include:

(a) Hypoglycaemia

(b) Hyperglycaemia

(c) Hypothalamic lesions

(d) Cystinosis

(e) Pituitary stalk lesion

3 Actions if vasopressin include:

(a) Decreased blood pressure

(b) Increased blood pressure

(c) Increased permeability of luminal collecting duct epithelium to water

(d) Dampens sympathetic drive

(e) Promotes fluid loss from the body

4 Vasopressin mechanism of action:

(a) Acts on three receptor types, viz. V_{1a}, V_{1b} and V_2

(b) Receptor V_{1a} mediates, amongst other actions, glycogenolysis and platelet aggregation

(c) Receptor V_{1b} mediates, amongst other actions, release of GnRH

(d) Receptor V_2 mediates water retention

(e) Receptor V1 mediates vasoconstriction

Chapter 36: Renin-angiotensin-aldosterone system

1 Renin:

(a) Is synthesized and stored in the tubular cells of the kidney

(b) Is released in response to a rise in blood osmolality or to hypovolaemia

(c) Converts angiotensin I to angiotensin II

(d) Converts angiotensinogen to angiotensin I in the kidney and plasma

(e) Has no enzymatic properties

2 Angiotensin II:

(a) Is a weak vasodilator

(b) Is inactivated by angiotensinase enzymes in peripheral capillaries

(c) Is considered the most potent natural vasoconstrictor known

(d) Is important in the regulation of arterial blood pressure

(e) Stimulates Na+ reabsorption by the kidney tubule cells

3 Other actions of angiotensin I include:

(a) Cellular proliferation effects in smooth muscle vascular cells

(b) Inhibition of aldosterone biosynthesis

(c) Acts on sympathetic presynaptic nerve terminals to promote norepinephrine release

(d) Inhibition of epinephrine release from the adrenal medulla

(e) Stimulation of α-actin production

4 Angiotensin II receptors:

(a) Exist as at least two subtypes, namely AT_1, AT_2, etc.

(b) AT_1 receptors are expressed exclusively by, for example, aortic and kidney cells

(c) Only T_2 receptors are expressed in brain

(d) There may be several subtypes of AT_2 receptors

(e) The AT_2 receptor may mediate cell death

5 In heart failure:

(a) Impaired cardiac output activates the renin-angiotensin-aldosterone system

(b) This results in peripheral vasoconstriction

(c) Accompanied by increased parasympathetic drive

(d) The physiological response includes enhanced Na^+ and water retention

(e) Thereby increasing pre- and afterload on the heart, thus exacerbating heart failure

Chapter 37: Endocrine hypertension

1 Clinically:

(a) Two main forms of hypertension are recognised, viz. essential and secondary hypertension

(b) Essential hypertension has a well-understood aetiology

(c) Secondary hypertension is often the result of endocrine disorders

(d) Endocrine hypertension usually results from aldosteronism or excessive catecholamine or glucocorticoid activity

(e) Clinical hypertension is an important risk factor for cardiovascular disease

2 Hypertension of adrenal origin:

(a) May result from a phaeochromocytoma

(b) Which is an acetylcholine-secreting tumour in the adrenal medulla

(c) A phaeochromocytoma occurs only in the adrenal gland

(d) It is treated both with α- and β-blockers and by surgical removal

(e) Is usually caused by viral infection

3 Hyperaldosteronism:

(a) May be primary or secondary

(b) Primary hyperaldosteronism results from excess renin secretion, while

(c) Secondary hyperaldosteronism results from an adrenal adenoma

(d) Primary aldosteronism promotes Na^+ and water retention

(e) And can be treated by removal of an adrenal tumour

4 Hypertension:

(a) May also originate from renal or neural disorders

(b) For example, through possible 'resetting' of brain set points for blood pressure

(c) Or because of obesity, or

(d) Depression, or

(e) Insulin resistance and hyperinsulinaemia

Chapter 38: Insulin: I The pancreas and insulin secretion

1 Diagnosis of Type 1 diabetes may include:

(a) Frequent, large volume urine passage

(b) Clinically low hypoglycaemia

(c) Presence of ketones and glucose in urine

(d) Weight loss

(e) Hyperphagia (overeating)

2 The human pancreas:

(a) Lies adjacent to the diaphragm

(b) Consists of acini cells, which secrete digestive juices into the duodenum, and

(c) Islet cells, which secrete insulin and glucagon into the bloodstream

(d) Is not essential for life

(e) Is not a true endocrine gland

3 Insulin:

(a) Is secreted by α-cells in the islets of Langerhans

(b) Consists of two linked polypeptide chains α and β

(c) Circulates predominantly as a dimer

(d) Is cleaved from proinsulin through the action of a converting enzyme

(e) Can dimerize

4 Insulin secretion:

(a) Is inhibited by glucose

(b) Is mediated through cellular uptake of Ca^{2+}

(c) Which triggers movement of insulin-containing granules to the cell membrane

(d) And insulin release from the cell

(e) And finally by reuptake by pancreatic cells of unused insulin

5 Nervous control of insulin releases involves:

(a) Inhibition of insulin release by the neurotransmitter acetylcholine (Ach)

(b) Stimulation of insulin release by sympathetic agonists, e.g. epinephrine acting on β-receptors

(c) Inhibition of insulin by adrenergic agonists. e.g. epinephrine, acting α-receptors

(d) Brain nuclei, where stimulation of hypothalamic ventrolateral nuclei stimulates insulin release

(e) Whereas stimulation of ventromedial areas inhibits insulin release

Chapter 39: Insulin: II Insulin action

1 Factors that may lead to hyperglycaemia include:

(a) Excessive cigarette smoking

(b) Obesity

(c) Hypotension

(d) Hypertension

(e) Hypercholesterolaemia

2 Insulin's mechanism of action:

(a) Is mediated by a cytoplasmic insulin receptor dimer

(b) Involves a membrane-bound receptor that belongs to a larger superfamily of receptor tyrosine kinases, and its structure consists of:

(c) Two alpha and two beta subunits

(d) The two extracellular alpha subunits bind insulin, and

(e) The two intracellular beta subunits, which span the membrane and have their own autophosphorylation sites

3 Insulin's important physiological actions include:

(a) Removal of glucose from the circulation

(b) Promotes formation of lipids from fatty acids

(c) Uptake of amino acids into liver and skeletal muscle

(d) Inhibition of lipoprotein lipase

(e) Stimulus for production of ketone bodies

4 Fat:

(a) Is a relatively minor source of stored glucose

(b) Is a relatively unimportant site of insulin action

(c) Is significant in the metabolism of ketone bodies

(d) Contains lipoprotein lipase, an important enzyme in insulin action

(e) Is a target for glucagon action

Chapter 40: Insulin: III Type 1 diabetes mellitus

1 Symptoms of diabetic ketoacidosis include:

(a) Metabolic acidosis

(b) Glycosuria

(c) Ketonuria

(d) Drowsiness and vomiting

(e) Hyperactivity

2 Insulin lack:

(a) Creates a profoundly anabolic state

(b) Causes failure of glucose uptake into the tissues

(c) Deprives the cells of an important energy source, resulting in:

(d) Glycogenolysis, gluconeogenesis and lipolysis, which results in:

(e) A profound alkalosis

3 Type 1 diabetes mellitus:

(a) Is an autoimmune disease resulting in the destruction of pancreatic α cells

(b) And an insulin deficiency

(c) Is more prevalent in peoples of North European origin

(d) Involves infiltration of pancreatic islets by activated cells of the immune system

(e) Which cause a destructive insulinitis

4 Treatment of Type 1 diabetes mellitus:

(a) Principally is the administration of parenteral insulin

(b) And the need for a special diet

(c) With regular, frequent and careful monitoring of blood glucose

(d) And treatment with human insulin

(e) Which is prepared using recombinant DNA technology

5 Complications associated with poor diabetic control include:

(a) Diabetic retinopathy

(b) Nephropathy

(c) Proteinuria

(d) Microalbuminuria

(e) Neuromuscular atrophy

Chapter 41: Insulin: IV Type 2 diabetes mellitus

1 Type 2 Diabetes mellitus:

(a) Is less common in obese people

(b) Is independent of ethnic status

(c) Is now the most commons form of diabetes

(d) Is characterized by insulin resistance and relative insulin deficiency

(e) Most commonly occurs in young children

2 Signs and symptoms of Type 2 diabetes include:

(a) Hyperglycaemia

(b) Relatively high glycated haemoglobin concentrations

(c) Lowered blood glucose

(d) Always ketoacidosis

(e) Invariably hyperphagia

3 Treatment of Type 2 diabetes aims to:

(a) Normalize and control blood glucose

(b) Increase concentrations of plasma lipids

(c) Reduce blood pressure if raised

(d) Weight reduction if necessary and regular exercise

(e) Persuade patients to adopt sensible diets and give up smoking

4 Lipid-lowering drug therapies include:

(a) Statins

(b) Antihypertensives, if needed

(c) Oral hypoglycaemic drugs

(d) Insulin if there has been a history of poor control of the diabetes

(e) Aspirin

5 Oral hypoglycaemic drugs include:

(a) Insulin

(b) Glipizide

(c) Gliclizide

(d) Metformin

(e) Glucagon

Chapter 42: Glucagon

1 Glucagon is:

(a) Biosynthesized primarily in pancreatic β-cells

(b) Cleaved from preproglucagon

(c) Derived (in humans) from the preproglucagon gene on chromosome 3

(d) Released together with GRPP

(e) Has a molecular weight of about 3.5 kDa

2 Glucagon secretion:

(a) Is triggered by steep rises in plasma glucose

(b) Is inhibited by energy substrates such as ketone bodies

(c) Is inhibited by insulin

(d) Is stimulated by several gut hormones

(e) Release may be controlled also by the brain

3 The effects of glucagon:

(a) Are essentially similar to those of insulin

(b) Include blockade of glycogen synthesis

(c) And the maintenance of short-term glucose blood levels

(d) As well as the conversion of amino acids to glucose in the liver

(e) Are lipolytic within the liver

4 The glucagon receptor:

(a) Mutation has been linked to Type 1 diabetes mellitus

(b) Is unique in having no mutated forms

(c) Does have mutated forms, notably associated with Type 2 diabetes mellitus

(d) Also binds insulin

(e) Notably has a glycine to serine mutation in exon 2

Chapter 43: Gastrointestinal hormones

1 The gut hormones:
  (a) Are synthesized in the clear cells of the GIT
  (b) This is because of their selective staining with gold salts
  (c) In humans, G17 gastrin occurs mainly in the duodenum
  (d) In humans, G34 gastrin occurs mainly in the stomach
  (e) Gastrins mediate HCL release in the stomach

2 Gastrin:
  (a) Is released mainly by dietary sugars
  (b) And also by foods
  (c) Release is also under autonomic control
  (d) Decreases motor activity in the GIT
  (e) Relaxes the pyloric sphincter

3 Cholecystokinin (CCK):
  (a) Is secreted mainly by I-cells
  (b) Release is inhibited by free fatty acids
  (c) Stimulates glucagon release
  (d) Inhibits release of pancreatic enzymes
  (e) Delays gastric emptying

4 Vasointestinal peptide VIP:
  (a) Is a strongly acidic polypeptide
  (b) Occurs mainly in the Gut
  (c) Is a member of the secretin family of polypeptides
  (d) Is not found in the pancreas
  (e) Is released during GIT relaxation

Chapter 44: Energy homeostasis: I Summary

1 The neuroendocrine system:
  (a) Is not implicated in feeding behaviour
  (b) Has no control over energy homeostasis
  (c) Is located principally in the hypothalamus
  (d) May be a target for treatment of obesity
  (e) Utilizes leptin as a chemical messenger

2 When considering energy stores:
  (a) Carbohydrates are the main energy stores
  (b) The body stores strictly limited amounts of fat
  (c) The brain utilizes only glucose as energy fuel
  (d) Epinephrine stimulates lipolysis
  (e) Insulin is the only hypoglycaemic hormone

3 The control of food intake:
  (a) Includes a hippocampus appetite control centre
  (b) In lower species includes a powerful regulatory input through leptin action
  (c) Includes the release of the hormone leptin from lymphocytes
  (d) In humans has a powerful psychological input
  (e) Which overrides pure endocrine control

4 Other factors that may influence feeding in humans include:
  (a) Blood levels of ACTH
  (b) Psychiatric problems such as anorexia nervosa
  (c) Genetic mutations
  (d) Cultural practices
  (e) Gender

Chapter 45: Energy homeostasis: II Central control

1 In lower species (e.g. rats):
  (a) Feeding behaviour is more strictly controlled by neuroendocrine and autonomic systems
  (b) Medial hypothalamic lesions block feeding behaviour
  (c) Activation of the paraventricular nucleus by NPY/AgRP-expressing neurones promotes feeding behaviour
  (d) POMC/CART-expressing neurones inhibit paraventricular/lateral hypothalamic centres, which are:
  (e) Activated by leptin, the satiety hormone

2 Which of the following are true?
  (a) POMC neurones produce pro-opiomelanocortin, which is:
  (b) Spliced other active peptides, including α-MSH
  (c) Which is thought to activate feeding behaviour
  (d) Signals from the hypothalamic feeding centres are relayed to the periphery via the nucleus of the tractus solitarius
  (e) Which also receives afferent signals from the gut

3 Orexins:
  (a) Mediate food-seeking behaviour
  (b) Are long-chain fatty acids
  (c) Are also known as hypocretins
  (d) Also appear to influence sleep/wakefulness patterns
  (e) Have neurones, which act autonomously, unaffected by other neural mediators

4 In humans:
  (a) Leptins govern, absolutely, all feeding behaviour
  (b) Leptin production is related to adipose tissue mass
  (c) Circulating leptin levels are strictly related to adiposity
  (d) Intermittent feeding behaviour is reflected in short-term changes in circulating leptin concentrations
  (e) Peptide PYY may be a medium term satiety factor

Chapter 46: Obesity: I Causes of obesity

1 Obesity:
  (a) Is associated with an increased risk of hypotension
  (b) Is associated with a risk of Type 1 diabetes
  (c) May cause sleep apnoea syndrome
  (d) May affect at least 300 million people worldwide
  (e) Incidence is increasing with wealth in society

2 Known causes of obesity include:
  (a) Insufficient advertising
  (b) Modern food additives
  (c) Aggressive marketing of inexpensive alcoholic drinks
  (d) Financial stress
  (e) Stable long-term marital relationships

3 Evidence for a genetic link to obesity includes:
  (a) High incidence of gross obesity in identical twins
  (b) The *ob/ob* mouse
  (c) Occurrence of familial obesity
  (d) Tissue unresponsiveness to the hormone leptin, e.g. the *db/db* mouse
  (e) Estrogen receptor mutations

4 Hormones implicated in the aetiology of obesity include:
  (a) Insulin
  (b) Growth hormone
  (c) Thyroxine
  (d) Testosterone
  (e) Glucagon

Chapter 47: Obesity: II Cardiovascular and respiratory complications

1 Medical problems associated with obesity include:
  (a) Depression
  (b) Colon cancer
  (c) Ligament and tendon injury
  (d) Gallstones
  (e) Back pain
2 Decreased levels of lipoprotein lipase results in:
  (a) Elevated serum triglycerides
  (b) Reduced HDL cholesterol
  (c) Hyperglycaemia, resulting in:
  (d) Decreased affinity of LDL for its receptor on macrophages
  (e) Decreased risk of coronary artery disease
3 Cardiovascular problems related to obesity include:
  (a) Left ventricular hypertrophy
  (b) Right ventricular hypertrophy
  (c) Diastolic dysfunction
  (d) Pulmonary hypertension associated with:
  (e) Sudden death
4 Respiratory complications of obesity include:
  (a) Sleep apnoea caused by:
  (b) Fat deposition in the neck resulting in:
  (c) A rise in arterial Pa CO_2 and
  (d) Sudden wakefulness and
  (e) Breathlessness

Chapter 48: Obesity: III Insulin resistance and endocrine complications

1 The metabolic syndrome:
  (a) Describes a range of metabolic disturbances in the same patient, including:
  (b) Hypotension
  (c) Insulin resistance
  (d) Hypertriglyceridaemia
  (e) Hyperinsulinaemia
  (f) Obesity
2 Obesity in about 50% of women is:
  (a) Associated with the polycystic ovary syndrome (PCOS)
  (b) Which is less severe in lean patients
  (c) Who exhibit less severe insulin resistance, but who may nevertheless contract acanyhosis nigricans (skin pigmentation),
  (d) Impaired glucose tolerance, and
  (e) Type 1 diabetes
3 Other endocrine causes of obesity include:
  (a) Hyperthyroidism
  (b) Cushing's Syndrome
  (c) Hypothyroidism
  (d) Impaired GH response to GHRH
  (e) Impotence
4 Strategies for treatment of obesity include:
  (a) Production of a negative energy balance
  (b) Education about diet
  (c) Prescription, under supervision, of appetite suppressant drugs

  (d) Physical exercise
  (e) Inhibition of pancreatic lipase

Chapter 49: Calcium: I Parathyroid hormone

1 Calcium is essential for:
  (a) Bone growth
  (b) Blood clotting
  (c) Maintenance of the transmembrane potential
  (d) Stimulus-secretion coupling
  (e) Cell replication
2 Calcium metabolism is regulated principally:
  (a) By thyroid hormone
  (b) By exchange between bone and extracellular fluid
  (c) By parathyroid hormone (PTH)
  (d) In the kidney and digestive tract
  (e) Through binding to plasma albumin
3 PTH:
  (a) Gene is located on the short arm of chromosome 10
  (b) Is secreted from the parathyroid glands, which are:
  (c) Located on the thyroid gland
  (d) Glands occur in all aquatic vertebrates
  (e) Is also called parathormone
4 For synthesis and secretion of PTH:
  (a) PTH is a cleavage product of pre-pro PTH
  (b) Cleavage of pre-pro PTH occurs in the bloodstream
  (c) PTH is secreted from the cell as the free unbound molecule
  (d) And secretion is through exocytosis
  (e) Secretion is controlled by plasma calcium
5 Physiological actions of PTH include:
  (a) Stimulates uptake of calcium into bone
  (b) Stimulates reabsorption of calcium in kidneys
  (c) Promotes calcium ionization
  (d) Stimulates a metabolic alkalosis
  (e) Inhibits bicarbonate reabsorption
6 In the pathophysiology of PTH:
  (a) PTH excess causes profound hypocalcaemia
  (b) PTH causes hypercalcaemia
  (c) Hypercalcaemia is often the result of parathyroid tumours
  (d) Surgical removal of tumours is usually advisable
  (e) Hyperparathyroidism may cause hypercalcaemia

Chapter 50: Calcium: II Calcitonin

1 MEN:
  (a) Is the acronym for Minimal endocrine neoplasia
  (b) Has two main types: MEN 1 and MEN 2
  (c) MEN 2 is associated with mutations on chromosome 11
  (d) Is further classified into MEN 2a and b
2 Calcitonin:
  (a) Is a hypercalcaemic polypeptide hormone
  (b) Is synthesized in thyroid parafollicular cells
  (c) Is synthesized as a precursor
  (d) Plasma levels rise sharply with low plasma serum calcium levels
  (e) Gene sensitivity is sexually differentiated, being more sensitive in males
3 Physiological actions of calcitonin include:
  (a) Potent inhibition of bone resorption
  (b) Has no actions on osteoclasts

(c) May be important in protecting calcium stores during pregnancy

(d) May be a satiety hormone

(e) Potent appetite stimulant in primates

Chapter 51: Calcium: III Vitamin D

1 Vitamin D:

(a) Is a mixture of cholecalciferol and ergocalciferol

(b) Biosynthesis is blocked by sunlight

(c) Is converted in the liver to 25-hydroxyvitamin D_3

(d) Is inactivated in the kidneys

(e) Biosynthesis is regulated partly by parathyroid hormone (PTH)

2 Regulation of vitamin D metabolism involves:

(a) The action of PTH

(b) Phosphate ion

(c) Growth hormone

(d) Serum lithium

(e) Serum Ca^{2+} levels

3 The vitamin D receptor:

(a) Is a transmembrane receptor using cAMP as second messenger

(b) Belongs to a superfamily of nuclear hormone receptors

(c) Is highly lipophobic

(d) Initiates de novo protein synthesis in the target cell

(e) Mediates increased osteocalcin synthesis

4 Physiological actions of vitamin D include:

(a) Increased uptake of calcium from bone

(b) Stimulation of osteocalcin biosynthesis

(c) Inhibition of calcium transport through serosal to mucosal gut cells

(d) Stimulation of calcium ion reabsorption in the kidney

(e) Mediation of skeletal muscle contraction

Chapter 52: Bone remodelling

1 Bone:

(a) Is one third calcium and the rest is water and collagen

(b) Is present mainly as crystalline hydroxyapatite

(c) Matrix is laid down in concentric layers

(d) The osteon is the unit of structure in compact bone

(e) The Haversial canal houses only nervous tissue

2 Concerning cell types in bone:

(a) The osteoblast is one of several cell types that produce bone

(b) The osteoblast originates in the bone marrow

(c) Osteoclasts inhibit resorption of bone

(d) Osteoclasts originate from precursors of the mononuclear/macrophage lineage

(e) Under the influence of interleukin I

3 RANKL:

(a) Is the acronym for receptor activator of NF-$k\beta$

(b) Is a member of the TNF ligand family

(c) Inhibits proliferation of osteoclasts

(d) Effects are modified by osteoprotegerin

4 Bone remodelling:

(a) Is the cycle of new bone deposition and bone resorption

(b) Is independent of systemic hormone action

(c) Requires and adequate supply of calcium phosphate

(d) Is a continuous process

(e) Cycle takes about 100 days

Chapter 53: Metabolic bone disease: I Paget's disease

1 Paget's disease:

(a) Is a chronic bone disease

(b) Affects mainly young women

(c) Most commonly presents with bone deformity and pain

(d) Produces a normal lamellar bone structure

(e) Affects mainly spine, sacrum and femur

2 Complications of Paget's disease include:

(a) Decompression of spinal cord

(b) Compression of cranial nerves, causing:

(c) Deafness

(d) Spinal stenosis in vertebral Paget's disease

(e) Carpal tunnel syndrome

Chapter 54: Metabolic bone disease: II Primary osteoporosis

1 Osteoporosis:

(a) Affects mainly elderly men

(b) Is associated with significant morbidity and mortality

(c) Is defined as a fracture from a fall of twice the patient's height

(d) In women primary osteoporosis results from age and estrogen deficiency

(e) Never occurs in men

2 The main phases in bone mass change through life include:

(a) Attainment of peak bone mass during post pubescent life

(b) Completion of bone mass consolidation after age 30

(c) Commencement of bone mass loss from the age of about 30

(d) Postmenopausal bone mass loss, which is:

(e) Mainly cranial

3 Predisposing factors include:

(a) Gender

(b) Ethnicity

(c) Maternal history of osteoporosis

(d) Polymorphic alleles of the vitamin D receptor

(e) Excessive exercise

4 Concerning the role of estrogen:

(a) Estrogen deficiency contributes to osteoporosis and

(b) Is not age-dependent

(c) Estrogen dampens osteoclast function

(d) Estrogen replacement is often prescribed in post-menopausal women and

(e) Acts by suppressing genes that express IL-1, IL-6 and TNF

Chapter 55: Metabolic bone disease: III Secondary osteoporosis

1 May be caused by (for example):

(a) Type 2 diabetes mellitus

(b) Smoking

(c) Immobility

(d) Hypothyroidism

(e) Glucocorticoids

2 Glucocorticoids may cause osteoporosis:

(a) Especially in trabecular bone of the axial skeleton

(b) Directly, by inhibiting replication of osteoblasts and

(c) Blocking apoptosis of osteoblasts

(d) Increased biosynthesis of osteocalcin
(e) Stimulation of synthesis of collagenase-3

3 Indirect actions of glucocorticoids include:
  (a) Promotion of calcium absorption in the GIT
  (b) Increasing renal excretion of calcium
  (c) Inhibition of ACTH secretion
  (d) Inhibition of growth hormone production
  (e) Depression

4 Prevention and treatment of osteoporosis involves:
  (a) Moderation or elimination of smoking and alcohol intake
  (b) Estrogen replacement therapy which:
  (c) Carries the risk of breast cancer in women over 50 years of age
  (d) Use of bisphosphonates

Answers

Chapter 1
1. b.d.e
2. b.d.e
3. b.d.e
4. a.c.d.
5. a.b.c

Chapter 2
1. b.c.d
2. b
3. a.b.d.e

Chapter 3
1. b.e

Chapter 4
1. c.d
2. b.c
3. a.c.e

Chapter 5
1. a.b.c.d
2. c.d.e
3. b.d.e
4. a.b.d

Chapter 6
1. a.c.e
2. b.d.e
3. a.c.e

Chapter 7
1. a.c.d
2. a.c

Chapter 8
1. b.c.d.e
2. b.d

Chapter 9
1. b.c
2. b.d.e
3. b.c.e
4. a.d.e
5. a.c.d.e
6. a.b

Chapter 10
1. a.b.e
2. a.c.d.e
3. c.d.e

Chapter 11
1. c.d.e
2. b.c.e
3. a.c.d
4. a.b
5. b.c.e

Chapter 12
1. a
2. a.c.d

Chapter 13
1. c.d
2. d.e
3. a.b.c.d.e
4. b.d.e

Chapter 14
1. b.d
2. b.c.d.e
3. a.b.c.d
4. a.c.e
5. b.d.e

Chapter 15
1. a.b.e
2. a.b.c
3. b.c.d

Chapter 16
1. b.e
2. b.d.e
3. b.d.e
4. a.b.c.d.e

Chapter 17
1. a.b.e
2. b.c.d
3. b.c.d
4. a.c.d.e

Chapter 18
1. b.c.d.e
2. b.c.d.e
3. b.c.d

Chapter 19
1. b.c.d
2. a.c.d.e
3. a.c.d
4. a.b.c

Chapter 20
1. b.c.e
2. a.b.e
3. b.c.d.e

Chapter 21
1. a.b.e
2. a.c.d
3. b.c.d.e

Chapter 22
1. b.c
2. b.c.e
3. c.d
4. a.c.e
5. b.d.e

Chapter 23
1. b.c.d
2. b.c.d.e
3. b.c.e
4. a.b.d.e
5. a.b.e

Chapter 24
1. b.d.e
2. b.c.d
3. a.b.d.e

Chapter 25
1. a.c.d
2. b.c.e
3. a.c.d
4. a.b
5. a.b.c.d.e

Chapter 26
1. a.c.e
2. b.c.d
3. a.c.d
4. c.d.e
5. a.c.d

Chapter 27
1. d
2. b.c.e
3. b.d.e

Chapter 28
1. b.c.d
2. a.b.e
3. b.d.e
4. b.d
5. a.b.e

Chapter 29
1. a.c.d.e
2. a.c.d

3. c.d.e
4. a.b.e

Chapter 30
1. b.d.e
2. a.c.d.e
3. a.d.e

Chapter 31
1. c.d
2. b.c.d
3. a.b.d
4. d.e
5. b.c.d.

Chapter 32
1. a.c.d.e
2. a.b.e
3. a.b.c.e

Chapter 33
1. a.c.d.e
2. a.c.e
3. c.d.e
4. b.
5. a.b.c.d.e

Chapter 34
1. b.c.e
2. a.b

Chapter 35
1. c.d
2. b.c.d.e
3. b.c.d
4. a.b.d.e

Chapter 36
1. b.d
2. b.c.d.e
3. a.c.e
4. a.b.d
5. a.b.d.e

Chapter 37
1. a.c.d.e
2. a.d
3. a.d.e
4. a.b.c.e

Chapter 38
1. a.c.d
2. b.c
3. b.d.e
4. b.c.d
5. b.c.d.e

Chapter 39
1. a.b.d.e
2. b.c.d.e

3. a.b
4. c.d.e

Chapter 40
1. a.b.c.d
2. b.c.d
3. b.c.d.e
4. a.b.c.d.e
5. a.b.c.d

Chapter 41
1. c.d
2. a.b
3. a.c.d.e
4. a.b.c.d
5. b.c.d

Chapter 42
1. b.d.e
2. b.c.d.e
3. b.c.d.e
4. c

Chapter 43
1. a.e
2. b.c.e
3. a.c.e
4. b.c.e

Chapter 44
1. c.d.e
2. c.d.e
3. b.d.e
4. b.c.d

Chapter 45
1. a.c.d
2. b.d.e
3. a.c.d
4. b.e

Chapter 46
1. c.d.e
2. b.c.d
3. b.c.d
4. a.b.c.e

Chapter 47
1. b.c.d.e
2. a.b.c

3. a.b.c.d.e
4. a.b.c.d

Chapter 48
1. a.c.d.e.f
2. a.b.c.d
3. b.c.d.
4. a.b.c.d.e

Chapter 49
1. a.b.c.d.e
2. b.c.d.e
3. b.c.e
4. a.d.e
5. b.c.e
6. b.c.d

Chapter 50
1. b.d
2. b.c.e
3. a.c.d

Chapter 51
1. a.c.e
2. a.b.e
3. b.d.e
4. b.d.e

Chapter 52
1. b.c.d
2. b.d.e
3. a.b.d
4. a.c.d

Chapter 53
1. a.c.e
2. b.c.d.e

Chapter 54
1. b.d
2. a.c.d
3. a.b.c.d
4. a.b.c.d.e

Chapter 55
1. b.c.e
2. a.b.e
3. b.c.d
4. a.b.c.d

Appendix: Normal Values

ACTH	0900 h	10–80 ng/L
Aldosterone (recumbent)		100–500 pmol/L
AFP		<10 kU/L
Cortisol	0900 h	140–680 nmol/L
	2400 h	<100 nmol/L
FSH	♂	2–10 U/L
	♀ Follicular	2–8 U/L
	♀ Postmenopausal	>15 U/L
GH	Post-glucose load	<2 mU/L
	Stress	>20 mU/L
Insulin	Fasting	3–15 mU/L
	Hypoglycaemia	<3 mU/L
LH	♂	2–10 U/L
	♀ Follicular	2–10 U/L
	♀ Postmenopausal	>20 U/L
PTH		10–65 ng/L
Prolactin		50–400 mU/L
Renin		13–114 mU/L
Testosterone	♂	9–30 nmol/L
	♀	<2.5 nmol/L
TSH		0.3–4.0 mU/L
Free T_4		9–26 pmol/L
Free T_3		3.0–8.8 pmol/L

Glossary

ABP: androgen-binding protein

ACTH: adrenocorticotrophic hormone

ADH: antidiuretic hormone (vasopressin)

adrenal hyperplasia: increased cell growth of the adrenal gland

amenorrhoea: absence or cessation of menstrual periods

anabolic: promotion of protein synthesis and tissue growth, e.g. use of anabolic steroids

androgen: steroid that stimulates male sex organ development and maintains male sexual function

apoptosis: programmed cell death

autosomal: genetic trait not originating from a sex chromosome

AVP: arginine vasopressin

CA: cyproterone acetate

carotinaemia: increased circulating carotene levels secondary to vitamin A deficiency

CCK: cholecystokinin

COC: combination oral contraceptive

cortex: outer layer of organ or structure

craniopharyngioma: brain tumour derived from remnants of the embryonic Rathke's pouch

CRH: corticotrophin-releasing hormone

cryptorchidism: failure of descent of testes into the scrotum

DAG: diacylglycerol

dermopathy: disease of skin

DES: diffuse endocrine system of the GIT

DHT: dihydrotestosterone

dimerization: combination of two protein molecules

diploid: cell has two sets of chromosomes

dysgerminoma: malignant tumour of the ovary, analogous to seminoma of the testes; may arise from primitive stem cells

dysmenorrhoea: painful menstrual periods

DOC: deoxycorticosterone

endometriosis: occurrence of endometrial tissue in other pelvic areas than the uterus

endoplasmic: intracellular membrane system

ER: estrogen receptor

euthyroid: normal thyroid function

FFA: free fatty acid

fibroblasts: flattened, irregular connective tissue cells

follicle: group of cells in functional unit, e.g. thyroid, ovary

FSH: follicle-stimulating hormone

gestation: pregnancy; intrauterine period for fetus

GH: growth hormone

GHRH: growth hormone-releasing hormone

glucagonoma: glucagon-secreting tumour

gluconeogenesis: new synthesis of glucose

glycogenolysis: glycogen breakdown

glycosylation: adding oligosaccharide side chains to proteins

GnRH: gonadotrophin-releasing hormone

GRP: gastrin-releasing peptide

haploid: cell has one set of chromosomes

HDL: high density lipoprotein

HLA: human leukocyte antigen system

HRE: hormone response element

HRT: hormone replacement therapy

hyperaldosteronism: syndrome resulting from over secretion of adrenal aldosterone by an adrenal tumour, resulting in hypertension

hyperprolactinaemia: persistently raised plasma prolactin levels

hypoglycaemia: low blood glucose

hypogonadism: impaired function of testes or ovaries

idiopathic: unknown cause

IGF-1: insulin-like growth factor-1

insulinoma: insulin-secreting tumour

IP3: inositol triphosphate

ischaemia: localized tissue death through oxygen lack

karyotype: paired arrangement of chromosome set ranked in size

leptin: protein endocrine hormone produced by adipose tissue; it acts on the brain to reduce food intake in animals

LH: luteinizing hormone

lipolysis: fat breakdown

LPH: β-lipotrophin

medulla: inner or central layer of organ or structure

metabolism: integration of biochemical reactions in the body

MSH: melanocyte-stimulating hormone

MCR-4: melanocortin-4 receptor

nephropathy: kidney disease or damage to kidney, causing impaired kidney function

neuromodulator: relatively prolonged-acting chemical released from a neurone

neuropathy: disease or damage to peripheral nerves caused by (e.g.) hyperglycaemia in diabetes mellitus

OC: oral contraceptive

oligomenorrhoea: irregular menstruation

oligosaccharides: linked reducing sugars (or monosaccharides)

osteoclast: bone-destroying multinucleate cell

phaeochromocytoma: catecholamine-secreting tumour; causes hypertension

PKA: protein kinase A

PKC: protein kinase C

PIP2: phosphoinositol

PLC: phospholipase C

primary amenorrhoea: failure of menstruation at puberty

progestational: eliciting progesterone-like responses

proteolysis: breakdown of protein

pseudocyesis: phantom pregnancy

PTH: parathyroid hormone

Rathke's pouch: embryonic structure contributing to pituitary development

renin: enzyme hormone released from the kidney into the blood by stress symptoms, e.g. in breast cancer

retinopathy: disease or damage to retina causing impaired vision or blindness, caused by (e.g.) hypertension

RNA: ribonucleic acid

scleroderma: autoimmune disease causing skin thickening and may attack other tissues, especially lungs

secondary amenorrhoea: cessation of established menstrual periods

SERM: selective estrogen receptor modulator

SHBG: sex hormone-binding globulin

T$_3$: tri-iodothyronine

T$_4$: thyroxine

TFT: thyroid function test

theca interna: estrogen-secreting cells of ovarian follicle

TNF: tissue necrosis factor

TRH: thyrotrophin-releasing hormone

trimester: defined 3-month period of pregnancy

trophic: causing growth

TSH: thyroid-stimulating hormone

ultimobranchial gland: calcitonin-producing avian gland

VIP: vasointestinal peptide

virilization: extreme result of overproduction of androgens by women, resulting in hirsutism, baldness, increased muscle bulk, voice deepening and clitoral enlargement

Index

In this index diagrams, photographs, tables and figures are indicated in **bold** type.